# TYPE 2 DIABETES

# *Your Healthy*
# *Living Guide*

## Tips, Techniques, and Practical Advice for Living Well with Diabetes

### American Diabetes Association

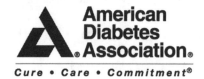

American
Diabetes
Association

*Cure • Care • Commitment*®

*Director, Book Publishing,* Robert Anthony; *Managing Editor, Book Publishing,* Abe Ogden; *Editor,* Rebekah Renshaw; *Production Manager,* Melissa Sprott; *Composition,* Circle Graphics; *Cover Design,* Michele de la Menardiere; *Printer,* United Graphics, Inc.

Printed in the United States of America
1 3 5 7 9 10 8 6 4 2

The suggestions and information contained in this publication are generally consistent with the *Clinical Practice Recommendations* and other policies of the American Diabetes Association, but they do not represent the policy or position of the Association or any of its boards or committees. Reasonable steps have been taken to ensure the accuracy of the information presented. However, the American Diabetes Association cannot ensure the safety or efficacy of any product or service described in this publication. Individuals are advised to consult a physician or other appropriate health care professional before undertaking any diet or exercise program or taking any medication referred to in this publication. Professionals must use and apply their own professional judgment, experience, and training and should not rely solely on the information contained in this publication before prescribing any diet, exercise, or medication. The American Diabetes Association—its officers, directors, employees, volunteers, and members—assumes no responsibility or liability for personal or other injury, loss, or damage that may result from the suggestions or information in this publication.

∞ The paper in this publication meets the requirements of the ANSI Standard Z39.48-1992 (permanence of paper).

ADA titles may be purchased for business or promotional use or for special sales. To purchase more than 50 copies of this book at a discount, or for custom editions of this book with your logo, contact the American Diabetes Association at the address below, at booksales@diabetes.org, or by calling 703-299-2046.

American Diabetes Association
1701 North Beauregard Street
Alexandria, Virginia 22311

**Library of Congress Cataloging-in-Publication Data**

Type 2 diabetes: your healthy living guide: tips, techniques, and practical advice for living well with diabetes. — 4th ed.
     p. cm.
  Includes bibliographical references and index.
  ISBN 978-1-58040-286-6 (alk. paper)
  1. Non-insulin-dependent diabetes--Popular works. I. American Diabetes Association. II. Title: Type two diabetes.

  RC660.4.T97 2009
  616.4'62--dc22
                          2008055048

# Table of Contents

# Foreword

*Type 2 Diabetes: Your Healthy Living Guide, Fourth Edition* has been updated and expanded to provide you with all the latest information you need to live a healthy life with diabetes. It takes you through the basics of what diabetes is, gives you tips on medical care, and how to make a plan to care for your diabetes. You'll learn about the newest meal-planning tools and medications and what's expected of you and your health care providers in monitoring your health. You'll find out how to steer clear of diabetes complications, fit diabetes into you lifestyle, and navigate your way through the emotional ups and downs of living with diabetes.

*Type 2 Diabetes: Your Healthy Living Guide, Fourth Edition* gives you the tools and techniques you'll need to help you meet the challenge of diabetes. By meeting the challenges you face, you will improve your diabetes control and your overall health. Be sure to ask your health care providers for help when you need it, and try your new-found skills every chance you get. Your reward will be your better health, today and tomorrow.

# Acknowledgments

*Many thanks to the reviewers of this book:*

Marilynn S Arnold, MS, RD, LD, CDE
Dayton Children's Medical Center
Dayton, Ohio

Virginia Peragallo-Dittko, RN, BC-ADM, MA, CDE
Director, Diabetes Education Center
Winthrop-University Hospital
Mineola, NY

Stephanie Dunbar, RD, CDE
American Diabetes Association
Alexandria, Virginia

# CHAPTER 1

# Introduction to Type 2 Diabetes

If you've recently been diagnosed with type 2 diabetes, you probably have a lot of questions. That's good—finding out more about the disease is an important step in learning how to manage it. Throughout this book, you'll learn about a lot of things you may not even have thought of yet—how to build a meal plan, how to deal with diabetes complications, and how medications fit into a care plan. But for now, let's talk about the basics. Here are some questions you may have—and some answers.

## WHAT IS DIABETES?

Diabetes is a chronic disease that affects your body's ability to change food into energy. Every part of your body needs energy to do its work, just like a car needs gasoline to run. That's why diabetes can make you feel tired or not quite yourself. Even if you feel fine, "running on less gas" affects nearly every part of your body.

Here's how it works: After you eat a meal, your body breaks your food down into many parts. One of those is *glucose,* a type of sugar. Glucose is the fuel that your body uses for energy.

Glucose travels to cells everywhere in your body through the bloodstream; however, glucose can't get into hungry cells without a hormone called *insulin*. Insulin is made by special cells called *beta cells* in an organ called the *pancreas*. Insulin is stored in the pancreas until it is needed. When glucose levels in your blood start to go up after you eat, the pancreas releases insulin to help glucose get into cells throughout the body. Think of insulin as the key that opens the door so glucose can get into the cells and make energy.

People with diabetes either can't make enough insulin, or their bodies can't use it effectively. Without insulin, glucose can't get into the cells, and the cells run out of energy. Over time, those hungry cells become damaged, and glucose builds up in the bloodstream, with nowhere to go.

There are two kinds of diabetes. In *type 1 diabetes,* the beta cells in the pancreas don't produce any insulin at all. This is why people with type 1 diabetes must replace insulin through injection to live.

*Type 2 diabetes* happens when the beta cells don't make enough insulin, or the body doesn't use the insulin effectively. A person with type 2 diabetes might add insulin over time, as one of many therapies.

Both types of diabetes can cause other health problems. Over time, the buildup of glucose in the bloodstream and the

## Diabetes in the U.S.

- 24 million people in the U.S. have diabetes.
- 90–95% have type 2 diabetes.
- 5–10% have type 1 diabetes.
- Nearly 8% of the total population has diabetes.
- 23% of people age 60 or older have diabetes.

Source: *Real-Life Guide to Diabetes* (ADA, 2009)

lack of energy supplied to cells can hurt your eyes, kidneys, nerves, heart, and blood vessels.

Type 2 diabetes is much more common than type 1. About 24 million Americans have diabetes and most of them—9 out of 10—have type 2.

# HOW DID I GET TYPE 2 DIABETES?

Researchers aren't sure what causes type 2 diabetes. They do know that you can't catch it from someone else, like you can the flu. They know it isn't caused by eating too much sugar. Type 2 diabetes is not a simple disease. You can't pinpoint the one thing that caused your diabetes, because it probably wasn't just one thing.

Type 2 diabetes usually comes on slowly. It was probably developing for years before you were diagnosed. Some people experience symptoms that warn them that something is wrong. Common symptoms include constant thirst; constant hunger; frequent urination; blurred vision; fatigue; tingling, numbness, or pain in your hands or feet; dry, itchy skin; and infections of the skin, gums, bladder, or vagina that keep coming back or heal slowly. But other people don't have any symptoms, and don't realize anything is wrong until their doctor tells them they have type 2 diabetes.

The only way to know for sure that you have type 2 diabetes is to have your doctor do a blood test. There are several tests doctors use; common tests include the *fasting plasma glucose test (FPG)* and the *oral glucose tolerance test (OGTT)*. If the test finds that the amount of glucose in your blood is too high, you have type 2 diabetes.

Doctors recommend that everyone get one of these tests regularly after they turn 45. That's because **age** is one of the risk factors for type 2 diabetes. (That's why type 2 diabetes used to be called *adult onset diabetes*.) But now we know that younger people, even children, can develop type 2 diabetes. So, it is important to consider the other risk factors, too.

Your **family** plays a role in your type 2 diabetes risk. If one of your parents, or a brother or sister has type 2 diabetes, you are more likely to develop it. African Americans, Latinos, Native Americans, Asian Americans, and Pacific Islanders are more likely to develop type 2 diabetes as well.

For many people, being **overweight** contributes to type 2 diabetes. When you are overweight, the cells in your body can't use the insulin your pancreas makes as efficiently. This is called *insulin resistance.* When you have insulin resistance, your pancreas works harder to make more and more insulin to try and move the glucose from your bloodstream into your cells. When your pancreas can't keep up, your blood glucose starts to rise. After years of working too hard, your pancreas may just burn out. (See "What's Your Body Mass Index?," page 6, to see if you are overweight.) The location of your excess weight also plays a role. If you have an "apple" **body shape,** carrying most of your extra weight above the belt, you are more at risk for diabetes, as well as for other serious health problems like high blood pressure and heart disease.

If you don't get much **exercise,** you may be at higher risk. Exercise helps use the insulin you have and can reduce insulin resistance.

People with **high blood pressure** and/or high levels of fats (or *lipids*) in their blood are also at greater risk for developing type 2 diabetes. **Cholesterol and triglycerides** are types of blood fats that doctors measure. These factors also put you at higher risk for heart disease, so it is important to try to lower them. (See Chapter 5 for more information on diabetes, cholesterol, and blood pressure.)

Women who get a temporary type of diabetes when they are pregnant, called *gestational diabetes,* are more likely to have type 2 diabetes when they get older. Also, women who have had a baby weighing 9 pounds or more are at greater risk for developing type 2 diabetes.

## Risk Factors for Type 2 Diabetes

You are more likely to have type 2 diabetes if you

- Have immediate family with diabetes
- Are overweight (BMI above 25)
- Are African American, Latino, Native American, Asian American, or Pacific Islander
- Are at least 45 years old
- Are not physically active
- Have impaired glucose tolerance (pre-diabetes)
- Have high blood pressure, low HDL, or high triglycerides
- Have had gestational diabetes or have delivered a baby weighing over 9 pounds
- Have a history of vascular disease

People can help control some risk factors, while others are out of their control. Now that you know you have type 2 diabetes, talk to your family about their need for screening, and encourage them to pay attention to other risk factors they can change.

# WHAT CAN I DO ABOUT MY TYPE 2 DIABETES?

There is no cure for diabetes. Your health care provider cannot give you anything to make it go away. It is a chronic disease, meaning that you will have to live with it the rest of your life.

The good news is you can learn to manage your diabetes. There will be many people to help you, like members of your diabetes care team; however, because nearly all of your diabetes treatments will be things you do yourself or decisions you make, it's important for you to know how to properly care for yourself. For example:

**Making healthy food choices** is one of the best things you can do to manage your diabetes. Because diabetes is about the body's ability to change food into energy, your eating habits are especially important.

## What's Your Body Mass Index?

One way to determine whether your weight is a risk factor for diabetes is to figure out your *body mass index,* or *BMI.* In general, the higher your BMI (over 25), the greater your risk for type 2 diabetes. To figure out your BMI, multiply your weight in pounds by 705. Divide this answer by your height in inches. Now divide that answer by your height in inches again. The answer is your BMI. Some BMIs are already figured out in the table below.

### BODY MASS INDEX (BMI)

| | 19 | 20 | 21 | 22 | 23 | 24 | 25 | 26 | 27 | 28 | 29 | 30 | 35 | 40 |
|---|---|---|---|---|---|---|---|---|---|---|---|---|---|---|
| Height (inches) | | | | | | Body Weight (pounds) | | | | | | | | |
| 58 | 91 | 96 | 100 | 105 | 110 | 115 | 119 | 124 | 129 | 134 | 138 | 143 | 167 | 191 |
| 59 | 94 | 99 | 104 | 109 | 114 | 119 | 124 | 128 | 133 | 138 | 143 | 148 | 173 | 198 |
| 60 | 97 | 102 | 107 | 112 | 118 | 123 | 128 | 133 | 138 | 143 | 148 | 153 | 179 | 204 |
| 61 | 100 | 106 | 111 | 116 | 122 | 127 | 132 | 137 | 143 | 148 | 153 | 158 | 185 | 211 |
| 62 | 104 | 109 | 115 | 120 | 126 | 131 | 136 | 142 | 147 | 153 | 158 | 164 | 191 | 218 |
| 63 | 107 | 113 | 118 | 124 | 130 | 135 | 141 | 146 | 152 | 158 | 163 | 169 | 197 | 225 |
| 64 | 110 | 116 | 122 | 128 | 134 | 140 | 145 | 151 | 157 | 163 | 169 | 174 | 204 | 232 |
| 65 | 114 | 120 | 126 | 132 | 138 | 144 | 150 | 156 | 162 | 168 | 171 | 180 | 210 | 240 |
| 66 | 118 | 124 | 130 | 136 | 142 | 148 | 155 | 161 | 167 | 173 | 179 | 186 | 215 | 247 |
| 67 | 121 | 127 | 134 | 140 | 146 | 153 | 159 | 166 | 172 | 178 | 185 | 191 | 223 | 255 |
| 68 | 125 | 131 | 138 | 144 | 151 | 158 | 164 | 171 | 177 | 184 | 190 | 197 | 230 | 262 |
| 69 | 128 | 135 | 142 | 149 | 155 | 162 | 169 | 176 | 182 | 189 | 196 | 203 | 236 | 270 |
| 70 | 132 | 139 | 146 | 153 | 160 | 167 | 174 | 181 | 188 | 195 | 202 | 207 | 243 | 278 |
| 71 | 136 | 143 | 150 | 157 | 165 | 172 | 179 | 186 | 193 | 200 | 208 | 215 | 250 | 286 |
| 72 | 140 | 147 | 154 | 162 | 169 | 177 | 184 | 191 | 199 | 206 | 213 | 221 | 258 | 294 |
| 73 | 144 | 151 | 159 | 166 | 174 | 182 | 189 | 197 | 204 | 212 | 219 | 227 | 265 | 302 |
| 74 | 148 | 155 | 163 | 171 | 179 | 186 | 194 | 202 | 210 | 218 | 225 | 233 | 272 | 311 |
| 75 | 152 | 160 | 168 | 176 | 184 | 192 | 200 | 208 | 216 | 224 | 232 | 240 | 279 | 319 |
| 76 | 156 | 164 | 172 | 180 | 189 | 197 | 205 | 213 | 221 | 230 | 238 | 246 | 287 | 328 |

Find your height in the left column. Move across the row to find your weight. The number at the top of the column is your BMI.

To find out whether you are overweight, compare your BMI to the figures below:

- A BMI of 20 to 25 is normal weight.
- A BMI of 26 to 30 is overweight.
- A BMI of 30 or greater is severely obese.

What you eat, when you eat it, how much you eat, and how you combine different foods can all affect the amount of glucose in your bloodstream. How much a food raises your blood glucose is based on the type of food, how it is prepared, how much you eat of it, when you eat it, and what you eat along with it. Over time, you can learn how to choose meals, portion sizes, and eating times that will help you keep blood glucose levels in a healthy range. The higher the quality of foods you eat, the more nutrients your body has to be strong and resist disease—just like everyone with or without diabetes. (See Chapter 3 for more information about planning meals.)

**Exercise** is another way to lower blood glucose levels. When you exercise, some of the glucose in your blood gets used up. It also helps cells in your muscles use insulin better, so even more glucose is removed from the blood. When you add exercise to your daily schedule, such as a 20-minute walk, you may lose weight, too. (See Chapter 3 for more information on exercise.)

Even if you are very careful about your eating and exercise habits, it is likely that at some point in the future you will need **diabetes medication.** Diabetes pills are medicine that lower blood glucose levels; however, they are not insulin. If changes in your eating habits, exercise, and diabetes pills do not lower your blood glucose enough, you may need to take insulin instead of diabetes pills, or you may need to take insulin along with diabetes pills. Your doctor will walk you through the options when, and if, changing your eating plan and exercise are not enough to keep your blood glucose in the target range. (See Chapter 4 for more information on medications.)

## HOW DO I KNOW HOW I'M DOING?

To see how your work is paying off, track your blood glucose levels with a blood glucose meter. A blood glucose meter allows you to check your blood glucose level by yourself at any time of the day. Using the meter regularly can help you see how meal

## Understanding Your Blood Glucose Numbers

The following goals are the ADA recommendations for blood glucose control

A1C: < 6%
Fasting and before-meal blood glucose: 70–130 mg/dl
1–2 hours after the start of a meal: < 180 mg/dl

choices and exercise affect your blood glucose level. Over time, the patterns you see can help you make decisions—what to eat, when to exercise, or how much medication to take—to help manage your blood glucose level. This knowledge can give you more flexibility in your day-to-day activities, too. You can change your schedule around—eat at a later time or exercise more than usual—and still keep your blood glucose levels on target.

Another way to check your progress is to have your doctor perform an A1C test (also know as a *glycated hemoglobin* or HbA1C test). This test measures the amount of *hemoglobin,* a protein found inside red blood cells. Hemoglobin's job is to carry oxygen from the lungs to all the cells in the body. Along the way, the red blood cells also pick up glucose in the bloodstream, a process called *glycating.* When there is a lot of glucose in the bloodstream, the hemoglobin molecules pick up a lot of glucose.

The A1C test is different from the blood glucose meter because it can measure your average blood glucose management over the past two to three months. That's because red blood cells live for about 120 days. So, if you took an A1C test on March 1, it would tell you how well you did, on average, with your glucose management in December, January, and February.

In people who don't have diabetes, about 5% of all their hemoglobin is *glycated,* or linked with glucose. In people with diabetes, the number is higher—as high as 25% if blood glucose levels are well above normal. People with type 2 diabetes should have an A1C test done twice each year or more. Your diabetes care team will let you know how often you should be tested.

Estimated average glucose (eAG) numbers are now being given alongside A1C levels by many health care providers. The eAG is an estimate of your average blood glucose derived from your A1C and helps to make the comparison between your blood glucose and your A1C easier to understand. The eAG recordings will be reported in mg/dl, just like a blood glucose result is recorded.

All three kinds of testing are important. The blood glucose meter lets you learn more about how your choices affect your glucose management, and helps you make day-to-day decisions. The A1C test lets you and your doctor see the big picture, to see if your glucose management efforts are working over time.

## I DON'T FEEL SICK. WHY SHOULD I DO ALL THESE THINGS?

Think of it this way: If you learn to manage your diabetes, it won't ever make you feel sick. You should be able to keep doing all the things you enjoy. But if type 2 diabetes isn't managed, it can cause serious health problems. Over time, type 2 diabetes can lead to diseases of the heart, blood vessels, nerves, kidneys, and eyes. These diseases are called *diabetes complications*. (See Chapter 5 for more information about diabetes complications.)

You can do something to lower your risk and possibly even prevent diabetes complications. Bringing your blood glucose levels into target range will stop or slow the damage to your eyes, nerves, and kidneys. This has been confirmed by two different studies—the 1998 United Kingdom Prospective Diabetes Study (UKPDS) and a 10-year study called the Diabetes Control and Complications Trial (DCCT).

## How Can I Protect My Family from Type 2 Diabetes?

If you have diabetes, your children, siblings, or parents may be at risk for developing it, too. There are ways to help protect them:

- Share your meal plan with your family. Prepare nutritious family meals that everyone can enjoy.
- Involve your family in your education. Encourage them to visit your diabetes care provider, dietitian, and other health care team members with you.
- Make sure your family members have regular checkups with a health care provider experienced in diabetes. There are tests that can detect markers for diabetes before it develops.
- Ask your family members to be your exercise partners. Set goals together, and help keep each other motivated.
- Work to achieve and maintain ideal weight.

# HOW WILL I LIVE WITH DIABETES?

You'll need some time to absorb the news that you have diabetes. You may feel overwhelmed by all you must do and remember. You are still healthy but may feel sad because you don't think of yourself as healthy now. You may feel angry and wonder "Why me?" You may feel afraid of having a low blood glucose reaction, or the thought of future complications. These and other strong emotions are all part of diabetes. (See Chapter 2 for more information about dealing with your emotional health.)

Knowing that these emotions are common may help you recognize and acknowledge them. Seeking support from your family, friends, other people with diabetes, your health professional, clergy, or a mental health professional may help.

As you go through life with diabetes, you will likely have days when you feel angry, fearful, and frustrated. Some days will be easier than others. That's okay. Just do the best you can at the moment, and start fresh each day.

# Your Emotional Health

Being diagnosed with diabetes can bring on many powerful emotions: denial ("I don't want to think about this"), anger ("Why me?"), depression ("I feel sad and hopeless"), guilt ("I must have done something wrong"), helplessness ("I can't cope with this"), or lowered self-esteem ("Something must be wrong with me").

These feelings are normal and common. Many people feel this way when they first learn that they have diabetes. These emotions can be part of the process you go through as you learn to live with diabetes. No matter how long you have had diabetes, these feelings will be present on some days more than others. Learning to acknowledge and manage these emotions is another part of managing your diabetes. Remember, your emotional health impacts your physical health, too.

## DENIAL

Many people go through some denial when they are first diagnosed with diabetes. You may think that your health care providers have made a mistake. You may wish it would all go

## How to Move Past Denial

- Understand that denial is part of the process.
- Find someone (a family member or friend) who will listen to you talk about diabetes and your emotional response.
- Tell your friends and family how they can help you deal with your feelings and take care of your diabetes.
- Join a support group for people with diabetes. Talking with other people who are dealing with many of the same issues can help. (See "Resources" at the end of this book.)
- Talk with a mental health professional.

away. You may tell yourself that you'll deal with everything later. If you've thought any of those things, then you've gone through denial.

At first, denial can help you adjust to the news of your diagnosis. Eventually, denial gets in the way. People who continue to deny how serious diabetes can be are less likely to take responsibility for managing their disease.

Often, people deny difficult things that they feel are out of their control. Realizing what you can control can help you get past those negative feelings. Managing your diabetes will put you back in charge and help you continue to enjoy your life.

# ANGER

Diabetes and anger often go hand in hand. You may be angry that diabetes has threatened your health and disrupted your life. You may be angry at the things you now have to do to manage your diabetes. You may be angry with yourself that your blood glucose numbers aren't in the ideal range. These are very normal feelings. The trick is to learn to recognize when you are getting angry, and to channel it in a different way.

If you are experiencing anger, it is a good idea to figure out what is making you angry and how it is best to solve the

## How to Handle Your Anger

- **Let it give you strength.** Think about how you can use the energy of your anger. Next time you get angry, you can use that energy in a positive way, like taking a walk.
- **Learn more about it.** Write down when you felt angry, who you were angry with, and why you felt angry. Try to understand what is making you angry.
- **Defuse it.** If you feel yourself getting angry, talk slowly, take deep breaths, sit down, and keep your hands down at your sides.
- **Let it out.** Vent your anger, calm down, and then return to the situation.
- **Make it trivial.** Ask yourself just how important it is. Some things are just too trivial to be worth your anger.
- **Laugh at it.** Find something funny about it. Sometimes laughter can push out anger.

problem. When you feel angry, it can be easy to take your anger out on yourself or on others around you, such as your spouse, family, or friends. Dealing with anger in this negative manner will keep you from fixing the problem. The better you understand your anger, the better you will be able to handle it.

# DEPRESSION

Depression is common among people with diabetes. You may feel alone or set apart from your friends and family because of the extra work you do to manage your diabetes. Perhaps you are saddened by the news that you have a diabetes complication. Maybe you're down because you've been having trouble keeping your blood glucose level where you want it to be. Feeling down once in awhile is normal, but feeling really sad and hopeless for two weeks or more might be a sign of chronic depression.

Depression can be caused by a physical illness. Check with your health care provider to see if there is a physical cause for your depression. If a physical cause is ruled out, you may

## Are You Depressed?

- Are things that used to be fun no longer fun for you?
- Do you have trouble falling asleep, wake up often in the night, or want to sleep a lot more than usual?
- Do you wake up earlier than usual and have trouble falling back to sleep?
- Do you eat more or less than you used to? Have you gained or lost weight?
- Do you have trouble paying attention or get distracted easily?
- Do you feel drained of energy?
- Do you often feel nervous or "antsy"?
- Are you less interested in sex?
- Do you cry more often?
- Do you feel you never do anything right or think that you are a burden to other people?
- Do you feel sad or worse in the morning than you do the rest of the day?
- Do you think you would be better off dead? Do you think about hurting yourself or committing suicide?

If you answered "yes" to three or more of these questions, or if you answered "yes" to one or two questions and you have felt this way for two weeks or more, you may be depressed. Talk to your health care provider. If you answered "yes" to the last question, get help right away.

want to see a mental health professional. This person may be a psychiatrist, psychologist, psychiatric social worker, or counselor. Treatment may involve counseling or antidepressant medication or both; research has shown that a combination of counseling and medication works best. (See "Resources," page 159.)

# GUILT

We can feel guilty for things we do and for things we don't do. If you have ever gone on an eating binge, quit an exercise program almost as soon as you started it, or neglected your blood glucose monitoring for a long time, you are probably well aware of how guilt can get tangled up in diabetes care.

## How to Steer Away From Guilt

- **Make changes one at a time.** For instance, don't begin a new job, start a new meal plan, and go on an exercise program all in the same week.
- **Make changes gradually.** For example, don't expect to start a walking program by walking 45 minutes each day. Begin by walking for 10 to 15 minutes every other day. Then gradually increase your walking.
- **Give yourself credit.** Perfect glucose levels are impossible even if what you are doing is perfect. For example, your blood glucose can be raised by surgery, injury, hormonal changes, growth, medication changes, and more.
- **Take stock of your successes.** We are quick to criticize ourselves when things do not go well. And many times we overlook our successes. Give yourself a pat on the back for what you are doing.
- **View setbacks as opportunities.** Setbacks only come to those who are trying to accomplish something in the first place. Use setbacks as an opportunity to re-evaluate your goals.

Sometimes, guilt may prompt you to get back on track and make some positive changes. But most of the time, guilt is harmful because it causes negative thoughts. Your self-confidence slips, and you give up trying to do anything. Recognize that the things you do to manage diabetes are choices that you have both the right and the responsibility to make. You must respect your own energy as well as your goals.

# SELF-ESTEEM

Self-esteem has a strong impact on every part of your life. You do better in your work, studies, and personal relationships when you feel good about yourself. You are more likely to go after—and get—what you want out of life when you have a strong sense of your own worth. Others are more likely to think well of you, too.

The way your parents, family, teachers, and friends treat you from the time you are very young colors your sense of yourself. You form a sense of who you are and whether you like yourself; however, self-esteem is not fixed. It changes as you grow and accomplish new skills. In fact, it changes from day to day. You may feel better or worse about yourself depending on things like:

- How you think you look that day
- How others respond to you
- Your physical well-being
- How prepared you are for the day's work
- Whether you feel hopeful or hopeless about the future

Your self-image may be affected by diabetes, too. You may see yourself as ill or dependent. You may think less of yourself or wonder if there is something wrong with you. Having diabetes can change your self-esteem in positive ways, too. The challenges you meet, and the decisions you make, may add to your self-confidence and sense of accomplishment. Your growing self-confidence may inspire you to make more changes in your life.

## How to Raise Your Self-Esteem

- Identify what would make you feel better about yourself.
- Consider ways you could make those things happen.
- Identify something you like about yourself each day. You might like the way you dress, the handiwork you do, the way you cook, the volunteer work you do, or the sports you play.
- Associate with people who are supportive and caring about you.
- Avoid or ignore people who constantly criticize you.
- Tell people directly what you want and what you need rather than hoping they will pick up on nonverbal signals.
- Compliment yourself each day.
- Compliment others. They may return the favor.
- Try to have a few enjoyable moments for yourself each day.

If none of these work, consider talking to a mental health professional.

## Learning to Assert Yourself

Some people find it difficult to talk about what they need. They may be embarrassed to be different or to have their needs conflict with those of the people around them. Some people simply find it difficult to call attention to themselves. Others fear the imagined consequences of speaking up for themselves.

Getting what you need for your diabetes can be a challenge in social situations, in any relationship, in the workplace, and in the health care provider's office. Being honest about what you need may make it easier for you. When you are direct and honest, you give the people around you ideas about how to help you. Try these basic assertiveness skills:

- **Learn to say "no."** A simple "No, thank you" says that you respect yourself enough to act in your own best self-interest. You also respect the other person enough to know that he or she will understand.
- **Be firm.** Decide what you need. Then find a way to get what you need or do what you need to do. For example, don't risk low blood glucose by waiting to eat just because no one else is eating.
- **Be considerate.** Some people may be uncomfortable when you take a blood sample for testing or inject insulin. Give your companions a choice about watching you do these tasks.
- **Maintain self-respect.** If you respect yourself, you will have no difficulty explaining your situation and asking for help when you need it.
- **Be direct.** Explain things simply to others. Ask for what you need.

# STRESS

Everyone has stress in their lives—it is unavoidable. But when you have diabetes, you need to understand how stress can affect your blood glucose levels and your overall health.

Today, we're likely to feel stressed because of traffic jams, deadlines, relationships at home and at work, or finances. But to the body, stress still feels like a physical threat. The body reacts to stress as if it were under attack and in danger. Scientists call this the "fight or flight response." When this happens, the body rushes to make stored energy available to cells, so they can get the body away from the danger.

## Understanding Your Stressors

- **What causes you to feel stressed?** What causes little or no stress for you may cause great stress for somebody else. Make a list of the people or things that stress you.
- **How do you react to stress?** Pay attention to how you react. People react differently, so learn to pay attention to how you feel when you're stressed.
- **How do you handle stress?** How you perceive a stressful situation determines how much stress you feel. You can handle stress in a way that makes you feel in control, or you can handle stress in a way that makes you feel better temporarily, but worse afterward.

For people with type 2 diabetes, this response may not work very well. When the body releases stored glucose for energy, there may not be enough insulin to handle it. Then the glucose builds up in the bloodstream.

The body's "fight or flight response" was intended to deal with short-term threats. But today, our sources of stress don't always go away quickly. Feeling stressed for days, weeks, or months can lead to high levels of glucose in the bloodstream.

Stress can affect blood glucose levels in another way, too. When you feel stressed, you may find it harder to follow your regular diabetes management plan. It may be harder to stick with your meal plan, exercise routine, and regular blood glucose meter testing. You may not sleep well. All of these things can affect your blood glucose levels, and your overall health.

For all of these reasons, it is important for people with diabetes to learn more about what causes stress in their lives and how they can learn to handle it.

## How to handle stress

Sometimes, people choose to handle stress in ways that are damaging. They may turn to alcohol, prescription medications, illegal drugs, nicotine, or anything they think might lift

## How Do You Handle Stress?

When you are under stress, which of the following do you do? Circle T if the statement is true and F if it is false.

|     |                                   |   |   |
|-----|-----------------------------------|---|---|
| 1.  | Have a few drinks                 | T | F |
| 2.  | Talk to a family member or friend | T | F |
| 3.  | Have a snack                      | T | F |
| 4.  | Call a friend                     | T | F |
| 5.  | Smoke                             | T | F |
| 6.  | Take a vacation                   | T | F |
| 7.  | Ignore my diet                    | T | F |
| 8.  | Work on my hobby                  | T | F |
| 9.  | Not talk to anyone                | T | F |
| 10. | Take a walk                       | T | F |

### SCORING

For odd-numbered answers, give yourself 1 point for every F.
For even-numbered answers, give yourself 1 point for every T.
If you scored 9 or 10, congratulations. You're skilled at dealing with stress.
If you scored 7 or 8, you're doing pretty well, but might be falling back on some
    unhealthy habits or not doing all you can to reduce stress.
If you scored 6 or less, the tips on dealing with stress, below, may help.

or calm them. Some choose to overeat. Any excessive behavior, even gambling or oversleeping, may be a way to try to get away from stress.

Few of these solutions work, and with diabetes, they can be harmful. Below are some positive ways to deal with stress and get back on with your life.

- **Take a deep breath.** Sit or lie down and uncross your legs and arms. Close your eyes. Breathe in deeply and slowly. Let all the breath out. Breathe in and out again. Start to relax your muscles. Keep breathing in and out. Each time you breathe out, relax your muscles even more. Do this for 5 to 20 minutes, at least once a day. If you're at work or away from home, seek out a quiet, private space—an empty conference room or a bathroom—to do these breathing exercises for a few minutes.

- **Stay active.** Exercise raises endorphins, which counter-act stress hormones. On your lunch or coffee break, take a quick walk around the block or around your office building.
- **Get a massage.** Put yourself in the hands of a licensed massage therapist.
- **Talk about it.** Find a good listener to talk to when something is bothering you. Consult a therapist or join a support group.
- **Try something new.** Start a hobby or learn a craft. Take a class. Join a club or a team. Volunteer to help others. Form a discussion group on books, movies, or whatever interests you.
- **Get away.** Go on a mini-vacation or overnighter, or take a long weekend. Form a baby-sitting cooperative with other parents so you can get out more.
- **Soak in a warm bath.** The most comfortable bath water is about the same temperature as your skin. Linger in the bath for 20 to 30 minutes. Add bubbles or soothing herbs if you like.
- **Say "no."** Especially to things you really don't want to do.
- **Prayer and meditation.** Get in the habit of spending some quiet time each day in reflection and mediation.
- **Laugh about it.** Have a hearty laugh every day. Seek out funny movies, funny books, and funny people.
- **Sleep on it.** Sometimes things look better the next day. Get your 7 to 9 hours of sleep each day.

## YOUR SUPPORT NETWORK

There is strength in numbers. You don't have to face the emotions and stresses of diabetes alone. Your family, friends, and health professionals can help.

## Your family

Learn as much about diabetes as you can, and share what you have learned with your family. First, each family member needs to understand what diabetes is, how it is managed, and how to handle emergencies. You can give them books, magazines, or pamphlets to read to help them understand, or have them visit a website, a class, or a support group meeting to learn more. Health care professionals can also help you explain diabetes to your family. You might want to invite a family member to come with you to your next medical visit or to attend a support group meeting with you.

Also, be sure to share your diabetes management goals with your family. Let them know why each goal is important to your diabetes care plan and to helping you feel your best. Explain how they can support and help you as you work to reach that goal. Ask them directly for the help and support you need. (See Chapter 3 for more information about diabetes care plans and goals.)

Remember, your family can't manage your diabetes for you any more than your health care team can. Your family can provide support and encouragement, which can make your work easier. They can be understanding and patient as you go through a lot of change, but the choices you have to make each day are up to you.

## Your friends

You can decide what to tell friends and how much to tell. Be sure your family knows to follow your guidance. But remember, the more your friends know about your diabetes, the better they will be able to help you. As with your family, you can use books, magazine articles, pamphlets, and websites to help teach your friends about diabetes and what it will mean for you. Tell your friends outright what you need from them.

## Progressive Muscle Relaxation

1. Close your eyes and breathe slowly and deeply.
2. Start with the muscles in your face, working your way down to your feet and toes.
3. Inhale. Raise your eyebrows. Tense them. Hold for a count of three. Relax your eyebrows. Exhale.
4. Inhale. Open your mouth and eyes wide. Then close your mouth and eyes tightly. Squeeze. Hold for a count of three. Relax your eyes and mouth. Exhale.
5. Inhale. Bite down on your teeth. Hold for a count of three. Relax your jaw. Exhale.
6. Inhale. Pull your shoulders up. Hold for a count of three. Relax your shoulders. Exhale.
7. Inhale. Tense all the muscles in your arms. Hold for a count of three. Relax your arms. Exhale.
8. Inhale. Tense all the muscles in your chest and abdomen. Hold for a count of three. Relax your chest and abdomen. Exhale.
9. Inhale. Tense all the muscles in your legs. Hold for a count of three. Relax your legs. Exhale.
10. Inhale. Tense all the muscles in your feet. Curl your toes. Hold for a count of three. Relax your feet. Exhale.
11. Inhale. Exhale any tension that may be lingering in your body. Breathe in energy. Take several more slow, deep breaths. Enjoy the relaxation.
12. Gradually open your eyes.

## Your mental health professional

A mental health professional can help you explore your thoughts, feelings, worries, and concerns about living with diabetes and other issues in your life. Therapy with a mental health professional can help you deal with your emotions, discover new approaches to old problems, make changes in your behavior, and learn new ways of coping.

Depending on your needs, you may want individual, couple, family, or group therapy. Group therapy can give you added support and a chance to support others. Sometimes it's easier to find solutions to your problems when you share them and hear about other people's solutions to similar problems.

Find a therapist who supports you. You may need to talk to several before it feels right. (See "Resources" at the end of this book for professional organizations that can make local referrals.)

CHAPTER 3

# Your Diabetes Care Plan

Planning is very important to diabetes management. But before you can plan, you need to know where you are headed. You need goals, or *targets*. Then you can plan out the steps you will take to get there.

Your diabetes care team can help you choose the targets you want to work toward. Just as every person is different, each person's targets and care plan will be different. Your targets may change over time as you meet goals and set new ones. The important thing is to choose targets that you feel good about and that you believe you can reach.

Once your targets are set, you can begin developing a diabetes care plan. Your diabetes care plan may include recommendations for eating, exercising, weight loss, and medication; advice on how to cope with the stress and emotional side of diabetes; a plan for taking care of your eyes, teeth, skin, and feet; and even a plan for when you are sick or pregnant. Your plan should help you make choices each day that move you closer to reaching the targets you have set.

Remember, your diabetes care plan is just a starting point. Any plan will need adjusting as your figure out what works best for you, and as your needs change.

## Aim for the Target

People with diabetes need to set goals, or "targets" to work toward. Targets established by the American Diabetes Association (ADA) are listed below. Your personal targets may differ. Talk with your health care team about the best targets for you.

| Marker | ADA Target |
| --- | --- |
| Blood glucose before meals | 70 to 130 mg/dl |
| Blood glucose two hours after the start of a meal | Less than 180 mg/dl |
| A1C | Less than 7% |
| Blood pressure | Less than 130/80 mmHg |
| LDL cholesterol | Less than 100 mg/dl, or 70 mg/dl for those with heart disease |
| HDL cholesterol for men | More than 40 mg/dl |
| HDL cholesterol for women | More than 50 mg/dl |
| Triglycerides | Less than 150 mg/dl |

# DEVELOPING MEAL PLANS

Most people with diabetes have a meal plan. You can work with a dietitian to make a meal plan that is right for you. A meal plan is based on:

- What you like to eat and drink
- When you like to eat and drink
- How your diabetes is treated
- Your weight goal
- How much flexibility and variety you want
- How often you monitor your blood glucose
- Your level of activity
- What exercises you do
- When you exercise
- Your overall health

- Whether you need medications
- Your family, cultural, or religious customs

A typical meal plan includes breakfast, lunch, dinner, and a bedtime snack. You should not feel hungry or deprived on a diabetic meal plan. In fact, your meal plan should be built with your favorite foods and eating patterns in mind. Remember, it's all about choices.

Scientists have learned a lot about nutrition in recent years. We know now that everyone—whether they have diabetes or not—should try to follow an eating plan that is high in fiber; is moderate in protein; and is low in saturated and trans fat and cholesterol. Research shows that this type of eating plan can help prevent heart disease and some types of cancer. It can also help you manage your diabetes. Your entire family can benefit from a new meal plan based on these ideas.

## Foundation of a meal plan

### Carbohydrate

Starches, fiber, and sugar are the three main kinds of carbohydrate. As explained above, the body needs carbohydrate to provide energy for cells. Starches and fiber also provide many important vitamins and minerals that the body needs to do its work. Fiber can only be found in starches.

There has been a lot of confusing talk about carbohydrate in recent years. It's true that carbohydrate are the main nutrients in food that cause your blood glucose to rise, but that doesn't mean that people with diabetes should avoid all carbohydrate. Both the amount and type of carbohydrate that you eat will affect your blood glucose, but the amount of carbohydrate seems to have more of an effect than the types you eat. As you'll see, there are different kinds of carbohydrate, and all of them can be part of your eating plan.

In fact, carbohydrate are the basis of a diabetic meal plan because they are the fuel that the body uses for energy. Starches include breads, cereals, pasta, rice, potatoes, corn, whole grains, dry beans, and peas. These starches have very little fat. Biscuits, croissants, muffins, and cornbread are examples of starches that are made into products with added fat.

Fiber, the part of plants that your body can't digest, is found in fruits, vegetables, whole grains, and legumes (beans, peas, and lentils). All are low in fat and calories and have no cholesterol.

*Whole grains,* meaning that the entire grain kernel is used, contain both starches and fiber. Grain kernels contain three parts: bran, germ, and endosperm. The soft endosperm contains starch; the germ and the bran have lots of valuable nutrients, and the bran also contains fiber.

Whole-grain foods are more nutritious than foods that contain only the endosperm, because they contain the vitamins, minerals, and fiber from the germ and the bran. Research has shown that eating whole-grain foods can help prevent some kinds of cancer and heart disease.

It's important to eat similar amounts of carbohydrate at meals and snacks each day to keep your blood glucose under control. Decreasing your carbohydrate level to an unhealthy level will probably not get your blood glucose back to normal, so try to keep your carbohydrate consistent, and talk to your doctor about adding a blood glucose–lowering medication to help keep your blood glucose under control.

## Foods That Contain Carbohydrate

- Starches: bread, cereal, pasta, and starchy vegetables
- Sugars and Sweets: regular soda, dessert, ice cream, syrup
- Nonstarchy Vegetables: lettuce, broccoli, carrots
- Fruit: apples, orange juice, raisins
- Dairy: milk and yogurt

## Protein

Protein is found in both animal and plant foods. The body uses protein to help build tissues and muscles, and to help transport oxygen to cells through the bloodstream. Some protein foods, like meats, poultry, eggs, milk, and cheese, are high in protein, but they can also be high in saturated fat and cholesterol. Research has shown that high saturated fat and cholesterol levels can cause heart attack or stroke.

Today, there are many protein choices that are lower in fat and cholesterol. Lean meats and low-fat milk, yogurt, and cheese are good choices. Most fish and shellfish are lower in saturated fat and cholesterol than meat, and also high in protein. Plants like legumes (beans, peas, and lentils), soybeans, nuts, and seeds are low in fat and calories, have no cholesterol, and are also a source of protein.

### Top Five Leanest Cuts of Meats

| Beef | Lamb | Pork | Veal |
|------|------|------|------|
| Top round | Foreshank | Tenderloin | Leg |
| Eye round | Shank | Sirloin chop | Arm roast |
| Shank crosscuts | Leg | Loin roast | Sirloin |
| Tip round | Sirloin | Top loin chop | Blade roast |
| Bottom round | Arm roast | Loin chop | Loin |

## Sodium

Many foods contain salt or sodium. The body does need a small amount of sodium to protect cells from drying out, and for different electrical reactions that happen in the body; however, the amount needed is so small—and salt is in so many foods—that it is almost impossible to not get enough.

In fact, most people get too much sodium. It is helpful for everyone to watch the amount of sodium they eat because sodium can contribute to high blood pressure. High blood pressure can increase your risk of heart attack and stroke. For a person with diabetes, it is even more important to control because diabetes can make you even more sensitive to sodium's effects.

Many foods that don't taste salty still contain a lot of sodium. Cheeses, salad dressings, cold cuts, canned soups, tomato sauces, and many other foods all contain sodium. Even if you never add salt to your food, you still may get more than the recommended amount of sodium.

Table salt, the type of salt in your salt shaker, is actually sodium chloride, which is about 40% sodium. So, one teaspoon of table salt contains about two grams of sodium. On food labels, manufacturers list the actual sodium content, not the amount of table salt. (See "Reading Food Labels," page 41.)

## ADA Daily Sodium Recommendations

- The ADA recommends limiting sodium to no more than 2,300 milligrams (2.3 grams) a day.
- Any food with 450 milligrams or more of sodium per serving is considered high in sodium.
- If you have high blood pressure, the ADA recommends that you keep your sodium to less than 1,500 mg per day.

### Sugar substitutes

Sugar substitutes have very few calories and will not affect your blood glucose level. Unlike sugars, they can be used in your meal plan without counting them as carbohydrate. Sugar substitutes include saccharin (Sweet 'N Low, Sugar Twin), aspartame (NutraSweet, Equal), acesultame potassium (Sweet One, Swiss Sweet, Sunett), and sucralose (Splenda).

*Sugar alcohols* are another type of sugar substitute often used in sugar-free candies, chewing gum, and desserts. Isomalt, maltitol, mannitol, sorbitol, and xylitol are examples of sugar alcohols. They provide about half the calories of sugars and other carbohydrate. Even though they are called sugar alcohols, they do not contain alcohol.

Sugar alcohols don't raise blood glucose as much as the same amount of other carbohydrate; however, they are not *free foods* like other sugar substitutes. See the box below to learn how to count sugar alcohols in your meal planning.

---

## Tips for Carb Counting and Sugar Alcohols

Sugar alcohols don't raise blood glucose as much as the same amount of other carbohydrate. To figure out the amount of other carbohydrate you should count for a food with sugar alcohols, follow these tips:

1. Subtract **half** of the sugar alcohol grams from the total carbohydrate.

2. Count the remaining grams.

For example:

> Serving size: 1 bar
> Total carbohydrate: 15 grams  —  Sugar alcohol: 6 grams
> One bar counts as 12 grams carbohydrate (15−3 = 12)

---

### Saturated fat and cholesterol

The two main kinds of fats in food are *saturated fat* and *unsaturated fat*. Saturated fat is found in animal foods like meat and dairy products. Saturated fats cause your body to make cholesterol and raise your cholesterol level more than anything else you eat. Trans fats are a type of saturated fat that is especially harmful (See "A Note About Trans Fats," page 32).

Most plant foods (fruits, vegetables, grains, and legumes) are low in fat. The fat they do contain is unsaturated. There are two main types of unsaturated fats: *polyunsaturated* and *monounsaturated*. Both can actually help lower your cholesterol level; however, even unsaturated fats should be used sparingly because fat is high in calories. Most people need only about 30% of their daily calories from all kinds of fat.

## A Note About Trans Fats

You may have heard about another kind of fat called *trans fat*. Most trans fats, or trans fatty acids, are made by scientists in a laboratory. (Trans fats also occur naturally in meat and dairy products, but the natural trans fats don't seem to be as dangerous as the man-made ones.) Trans fats are created when liquid fats are turned into solid fats, which keeps them fresh longer. Food manufacturers sometimes add trans fats to foods to increase their shelf life—the amount of time between when they were made and when they would spoil.

In recent years, we've learned that trans fats are very dangerous to our health. Trans fats have the same number of calories as other fats, but they can raise cholesterol levels even more than saturated fats. That's because trans fats raise your LDL, or "bad" cholesterol, and also lower your HDL, or "good" cholesterol. High total cholesterol, high LDL, and low HDL all increase your risk of heart disease.

Everyone should avoid trans fats, but people with diabetes should look extra-carefully for trans fats in the foods they eat, because people with diabetes already have a higher risk of developing heart disease. Eating trans fats just multiplies that risk.

Many food manufacturers have removed trans fats from the foods they make. Some cities have even passed laws saying that restaurants can't use trans fats in their cooking, but trans fats are still out there. Most food labels now include a line for trans fats. Also check the ingredients list: If it includes "hydrogenated oils" or "partially hydrogenated oils," it contains some trans fats.

Trans fats are most often found in fried foods like French fries and onion rings, snack foods like chips, and baked goods. Many stick margarines and shortenings also contain trans fats. There is no recommended limit for trans fat intake—your best bet is to eliminate them as much as possible.

# MEAL-PLANNING TOOLS

Now that you know the basics of an eating plan, the next step is to learn how to plan meals that fit into your eating plan. Meal-planning tools like the food pyramid, carbohydrate counting, and exchanges/choices lists can help you make choices that support your plan and your targets. After you learn more about each tool, you can choose the one that best fits your lifestyle and eating plan.

As we've learned more about nutrition and health over the years, guidelines for food choices have changed. Many of

## Tips to Lower Fat and Cholesterol in Cooking

- Use nonstick cookware so you won't need to use as much fat.
- Cook food in a tablespoon or less of an unsaturated oil, such as olive or canola oil.
- Use nonstick vegetable oil spray, wine, or low-fat or nonfat broth instead of oils.
- Roast, grill, or broil meats on a rack so the fat drains off and away from the food.
- Drain the fat as it cooks out of meats when pan-frying.
- Baste with broth or wine rather than with pan drippings.
- Marinate meats and vegetables in lemon juice, lime juice, sherry, wine, vinegar, low-fat or non-fat broth, or vegetable juice instead of oil. Marinate in herbs and spices, which add flavor with little or no fat or calories.
- Microwave onions, garlic, peppers, and other vegetables in a bit of water instead of sautéing them in oil.
- Skim the fat from soups, stews, broths, gravies, and sauces. Chilling the food in the refrigerator until the fat floats on top and hardens makes the fat easier to remove.

us grew up learning about the *four basic food groups*. In the 1990s, this was replaced by the *Food Pyramid,* which divided foods into six groups and stacked them in the shape of a triangle. Then in 2005, the pyramid was revised to create a more flexible tool based on the number of calories a person needs in a day. The new system, called *MyPyramid,* also encourages regular exercise.

These eating guidelines are issued by the U.S. Department of Agriculture (USDA). The information is designed to help many different kinds of people. To help people with diabetes, The American Dietetic Association and the ADA worked together to create a pyramid tool specifically for people with diabetes. It is called the *Diabetes Food Pyramid.*

Like the USDA Pyramid, the Diabetes Food Pyramid divides foods into six groups: breads, grains, and other starches; vegetables; fruits; milk; meat, meat substitutes, and other proteins; and fats, oils, and sweets. You can see how these groups match up with the recommendations from the beginning of this chapter. Breads, grains, and other starches get the biggest block in the pyramid, at the bottom. Then the other groups stack up, with blocks getting smaller toward the top. The size of the block tells you how many servings you should be eating each day from those groups: The larger the block, the larger the number of daily servings.

The right number of daily servings for you depends on the calories you need, age, whether you are a man or a woman, and how much exercise you get each day. That's why the Diabetes Food Pyramid gives a range of servings for each group (See chart below). If you eat the minimum number of servings in each group, you'll be close to 1,600 calories a day. If you eat the maximum number of servings in each group, you'll be close to 2,800 calories a day. In general, most women follow plans closer to the minimum number of servings, while most men use a number of servings in the middle or high end of the range. A dietitian or nutritionist can help you figure out the best plan for you.

Once you've determined the number of servings you should eat each day from each group, then you can decide how to divide those servings into meals and snacks. When

## General Serving Guidelines

| # of servings | Breads, grains, & other starches | Vegetables | Fruits | Milk | Meat, meat substitutes and other proteins | Fats, oils, and sweets | Daily calorie intake |
|---|---|---|---|---|---|---|---|
| Minimum | 6 | 3 | 2 | 2 | 4 oz. | Sparingly | About 1,600 |
| Maximum | 11 | 5 | 4 | 3 | 6 oz. | Sparingly | About 2,800 |

planning your meals and snacks, remember to try lots of different foods from each food group along with foods from different groups at each meal. For example, eat many different vegetables, instead of getting stuck on one or two. This will help you get all the nutrients you need from your food and help keep you from getting bored with your eating plan, too.

When using the Diabetes Food Pyramid, it's important to know the serving size for each type of food. For example, one half of an English muffin is one serving—if you eat the whole English muffin, count it as two servings from the breads, grains, and other starches group. Below are some guidelines for serving sizes of common foods.

## Servings Sizes for Common Foods

| Food Group | Foods | One Serving Equals: |
|---|---|---|
| Breads, Grains, and Other Starches | Bread; cereal; rice; pasta; starchy vegetables like potatoes, peas, and corn; beans like black-eyed peas, kidney beans, and pinto beans. These foods contain mostly carbohydrate. Starchy vegetables and beans are in this group because one serving of them contains about as much carbohydrate as one slice of bread. | 1 slice of bread<br>1/4 of a bagel (1 oz.)<br>1/2 an English muffin or pita<br>1 6-inch tortilla<br>1/4 cup dry cereal<br>1/2 cup cooked cereal<br>1/2 cup potato, yam, peas, corn, or cooked beans<br>1 cup winter squash<br>1/3 cup rice or pasta |
| Vegetables | Spinach, chicory, sorrel, Swiss chard, broccoli, cabbage, bok choy, Brussels sprouts, cauliflower, kale, carrots, tomatoes, cucumbers, and lettuce. Starchy vegetables like potatoes, corn, peas, and lima beans are counted in the Breads, Grains, and Other Starches group, above. | 1 cup raw vegetables<br>1/2 cup cooked vegetables |

*(continued)*

## Servings Sizes for Common Foods (Continued)

| Food Group | Foods | One Serving Equals: |
|---|---|---|
| Fruits | Blackberries, cantaloupe, strawberries, oranges, apples, bananas, peaches, pears, apricots, and grapes | 1/2 cup canned fruit<br>1 small fresh fruit<br>2 tablespoons dried fruit (like raisins)<br>1 cup melon or raspberries<br>1 1/4 cup whole strawberries |
| Milk | Milk, yogurt | 1 cup non-fat or low-fat milk<br>1 cup yogurt |
| Meat, Meat Substitutes, and Other Proteins | Beef, chicken, turkey, fish, eggs, tofu, cheese, cottage cheese, and peanut butter | 1 ounce of meat<br>1 egg<br>1/4 cup cottage cheese<br>1 tablespoon peanut butter<br>1/2 cup tofu |
| Fats, Sweets, and Alcohol | Potato chips, candy, cookies, cakes, fried foods, and ice cream | 1/2 cup ice cream<br>1 small cupcake<br>2 small cookies |

## Carbohydrate counting

When you eat a meal or snack, it is usually a mixture of carbohydrate, protein, and fat; however, your body changes the carbohydrate into glucose faster than the protein and fat. Your blood glucose level goes up because of the carbohydrate portion. So, keeping track of how much carbohydrate you have eaten can give you an idea of how high your blood glucose is going to go.

With the carbohydrate counting tool, you count foods that are mostly carbohydrate. These include starches (breads, cereals, pasta), fruits and fruit juices, vegetables, milk, yogurt, ice cream, and sugars (honey, syrup). You do not count meats, fats, and most vegetables, because these foods have very little carbohydrate in them.

There are two types of carbohydrate counting: basic and advanced. Basic carb counting works best for people with type 2 diabetes who don't take any diabetes medications, or who take low dosages of insulin and/or diabetes medication. Advanced carb counting is better for people who take three to four shots of insulin a day or use an insulin pump.

In **basic carb counting,** the goal is to eat about the same amount of carbohydrate at about the same time each day. This helps to keep your blood glucose level in your target range throughout the day. Instead of counting exact grams of carbohydrate in each food, basic carb counting tracks the number of carb servings you eat each day. On average, one serving of carbohydrate-containing food has about 15 grams of carbohydrate. Some people find it easier to count carbohydrate servings than to count grams.

As explained above, **advanced carb counting** is more often used by people who take insulin and other diabetes medications frequently. That's because the dosage of insulin you take before a meal can change depending on how much carbohydrate you plan to eat. It's very important for these people to count their carbohydrate grams very carefully. So, people using advanced carb counting track the exact grams of carbohydrate in the foods they eat.

To use carb counting, you'll need a few tools. You'll need a kitchen scale, measuring cups, and measuring spoons to help you know how much you are eating. These tools will help you to accurately count the carbohydrate you eat. You'll also need a notebook to write down what you ate, how much of it you ate, and how many grams of carbohydrate it contained. Over time, this will help you build your own list of the carbohydrate content in foods you eat often, making it even easier to work carb counting into your daily life.

You'll also need some reference to tell you how many grams of carbohydrate are in different foods. There are several ways to get this information. Packaged foods will have the number of carbohydrate grams printed on the food label. (See "Reading Food Labels," page 41.) There are also books and pamphlets available that list the carbohydrate content of many foods; the ADA offers several. If you work with a dietitian or a nutritionist, he or she will also have resources on carb counting.

Carb counting also requires that you monitor your blood glucose regularly, so that you can make sure your eating plan is working. (See Chapter 4 for information on self-monitoring your blood glucose levels.)

Each person using the carb counting tool will have a different daily goal. The number depends on your age, whether you are a man or a woman, how much exercise you usually get in a day, and the other targets you've set. To learn more about how to set your daily carbohydrate goal, talk with a dietitian, or read *Complete Guide to Carb Counting,* by Hope S. Warshaw, MMSc, RD, CDE, BC-ADM, and Karmeen Kulkiarni, MS, RD, CDE, BC-ADM (ADA, 2004).

## Daily Carbohydrate Recommendations

The Dietary Guidelines for Americans recommend that people get 45 to 65% of their daily calories from carbohydrate. However, there is no set amount of carbohydrate that is right for everyone. The amount you need is based on several factors.

- Your height and weight
- Your usual food habits and daily schedule
- The foods you like to eat
- The amount of physical activity you do
- Your health status and diabetes goals
- The diabetes medications you take and the times that you take them
- Your blood glucose–monitoring results

Source: *Complete Guide to Carb Counting* (ADA, 2004)

# Exchanges/choices

Exchange lists are lists of foods grouped together because they are alike. One serving of any of the foods on a list has about the same amount of carbohydrate, protein, fat, and calories. Any food on a list may be "exchanged" or traded for any other food on the same list. In 2008, the exchange lists were revised in *Choose Your Foods: Exchange Lists for Diabetes,* making the system even easier to follow.

As with carb counting, the number of food exchanges/ choices planned for each meal and snack will be different for different people. It depends on your age, whether you are a man or a woman, how much exercise you get, and your targets.

To use exchanges/choices for meal planning, you'll need a kitchen scale, measuring cups, and measuring spoons so you know how much you're eating. You'll also need a notebook to keep track of what you eat, how much of it you eat, and how many exchanges it represents.

Exchanges/choices lists are available through certified diabetes educators and dietitians. These professionals can help you figure out an exchange plan that will help you meet your targets and help you learn more about exchanges. Your meal plan can be adjusted to fit changes in your lifestyle, such as work, school, or travel. Make sure to check your blood glucose frequently whenever you change your meal plan to see how different foods will affect your blood glucose level.

One thing to keep in mind: The serving size on a food label may not be the same as the serving size of an exchange/ choice. (See "Reading Food Labels," page 41.) For example, the label may say the serving size of fruit juice is one cup, but the exchange/choices list says the serving size of fruit juice is 1/2 cup. If you drink one cup of fruit juice, you need to count two fruit exchanges, not one.

## Choose Your Foods: Exchange Lists for Diabetes

The new system breaks the foods down into 16 groups:

*Carbohydrate*
1. Starch List
2. Fruit List
3. Milk List
4. Other Carbohydrate List
5. Nonstarchy Vegetable List

*Meat and Meat Substitutes*
6. Lean List
7. Medium-Fat List
8. High-Fat List
9. Plant-Based Proteins

*Fats*
10. Monounsaturated Fats List
11. Polyunsaturated Fats List
12. Saturated Fats List

*Other Lists*
13. Free Foods List
14. Combination Foods List
15. Fast Foods List
16. Alcohol

## Plate method

The plate method is a relatively new concept in meal planning and is starting to be used as a common meal-planning method because of how easy it is to use. It was first brought to light in the early 1990s by a group of dietitians. The concept is simple: Assemble healthy meals in the correct proportions, and spread the carbohydrate content evenly across the meal.

One of the best features about the plate method is that it doesn't require measuring cups, scales, or any other additional tools. All you need is a normal 9-inch dinner plate. When you're deciding how much to eat, imagine that the plate is divided into 4 parts, or quarters.

For both lunch and dinner, 1/2 of the plate should be filled with nonstarchy vegetables (tomatoes, onions, peppers, celery broccoli), 1/4 of the plate should be filled with starches (rice, bread, pasta, potatoes), and 1/4 of the plate should be filled with protein-rich foods (eggs, meat, cheese, fish, poultry). It is also recommended that you include one serving (8-ounce cup) of milk and one serving (small to medium-sized piece) of fruit along with your meal.

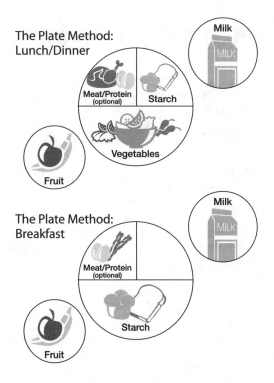

The plate method offers a lot of flexibility and allows you to eat in restaurants or anywhere else, as long as you fill your plate with the approved proportions. For more information, visit *www.platemethod.com.*

## READING FOOD LABELS

No matter what meal planning tool you use, you'll need to know what nutrients are in the foods you buy. Most foods have a "Nutrition Facts" box printed on their label that can tell you what you need to know. (See Nutrition Facts, page 42.)

The Nutrition Facts label includes a lot of information. For your meal planning, you'll want to pay the most attention to the serving size, the number of grams (or milligrams) of the various nutrients, % daily value, and the ingredients list.

# Nutrition Facts

**Serving Size** 1 cup (228g)
**Servings Per Container** 2

**Amount Per Serving**

**Calories** 260      **Calories from Fat** 120

| | % Daily Value* |
|---|---:|
| **Total Fat** 13 g | **20%** |
| Saturated Fat 5g | **25%** |
| *Trans* Fat 2g | |
| **Cholesterol** 30 mg | **10%** |
| **Sodium** 660mg | **28%** |
| **Total Carbohydrate** 31 g | **10%** |
| Dietary Fiber 0g | **0%** |
| Sugars 5g | |
| **Protein** 5g | |

| Vitamin A 4% | • | Vitamin C 2% |
|---|---|---|
| Calcium 15% | • | Iron 4% |

*Percent Daily Values are based on a 2,000 calorie diet. Your Daily Values may be higher or lower depending on your calorie needs.

| | Calories: | 2,000 | 2,500 |
|---|---|---|---|
| Total Fat | Less than | 65g | 80g |
| Sat Fat | Less than | 20g | 25g |
| Cholesterol | Less than | 300mg | 300mg |
| Sodium | Less than | 2,400mg | 2,400mg |
| Total Carbohydrate | | 300g | 375g |
| Dietary Fiber | | 25g | 30g |

Calories per gram:
Fat 9  •  Carbohydrate 4  •  Protein 4

## Serving size

The serving size information is found right under the "Nutrition Facts" headline. The serving sizes are meant to be close to what people actually eat—but you might be surprised. One serving may be a box, half the box, or three pieces. The label also gives the number of servings per container.

## Number of grams

Right under the calories and the calories from fat, the label lists the grams of total fat, saturated fat, trans fat, cholesterol, sodium, total carbohydrate, dietary fiber, sugars, and protein in a serving. Some foods may list other nutrients, too. Next to each nutrient is a number, followed by either "g" or "mg." These numbers tell you how many grams (g) or milligrams (mg) of that nutrient are found in one serving of that food.

This information can help you with carb counting, or keep you in line with goals like lowering your sodium or cholesterol intake. Remember to check the serving size; if you eat more or less than the serving size shown on the label, you'll need to adjust the number of grams or milligrams of the various nutrients. For example, if 1/2 cup contains 15 grams of carbohydrate, and you eat one cup, you need to count 30 grams of carbohydrate for that meal.

## % daily value

The label also includes a "% Daily Value" or "% DV" column. This tells you how much one serving of the food gives you toward the daily recommendation for that nutrient. The daily recommendations are set by the FDA. For example, the FDA recommends that adults get 1,000 milligrams of calcium each day; one cup of 1% milk provides 300 mg, or 30%, of that daily value.

You don't need to know all the recommended daily values when you shop. Just focus on the nutrients that you are targeting in your meal plan. As a general rule, it's a good idea to choose foods that are low in saturated fats, trans fats, cholesterol, and sodium, and/or high in fiber, vitamins, and minerals. Five percent or less of the daily value is low; while 20% or more is high. (See chart on next page.)

| Keep These Low: | Look for More of These: |
| --- | --- |
| • saturated fats | • fiber |
| • *trans* fats | • vitamins A and C |
| • cholesterol | • calcium, potassium, |
| • sodium | magnesium, and iron |

*Use the % Daily Value (DV) column when possible: 5% DV or less is low, 20% DV or more is high.*
*From http://www.nutrition.gov/index.php?mode=whole_story&story_id=161*

## Ingredients list

The ingredients list can also be helpful. Ingredients are listed by amount, so the main ingredient is listed first. For example, in bread, flour is usually listed first, and other things like oil and salt are listed at the end. It pays to read the ingredients list, because claims on packages can be misleading.

To use the nutrient information on the Nutrition Facts label, you need to know how much or how little of each nutrient you should be getting each day. It's difficult to track your daily intake of every one of these nutrients. Based on your goals and targets, you may want to pick two or three to focus on. For example, your goals may include reducing your sodium intake to lower your blood pressure; reducing total fat to help you lose weight; and using the carb counting tool to manage your blood glucose level.

The chart below can help you figure out how much of each nutrient you should be taking each day. The recommendations correspond to a total daily calorie level. So, if your meal plan aims to provide you with 1,500 calories a day, you should also shoot for taking in 300 mg of cholesterol a day or less. If you have one serving (one cup) of the food represented by the food label above, that would provide 30 grams toward your daily 300 grams. You can track the numbers with all

## Daily Values for 1,200- to 2,500-Calorie Meal Plans

| Daily Values | Calories Per Day | | | | | |
|---|---|---|---|---|---|---|
| | 1,200 | 1,500 | 1,800 | 2,000 | 2,200 | 2,500 |
| Total Fat (g) | 40 | 50 | 60 | 67* | 73 | 83* |
| Saturated Fat (g) | 13 | 17 | 20 | 22* | 24 | 28* |
| Cholesterol (mg) | 200 | 200 | 200 | 200 | 200 | 200 |
| Sodium (mg) | 2,300 | 2,300 | 2,300 | 2,300 | 2,300 | 2,300 |
| Potassium (mg) | 3,500 | 3,500 | 3,500 | 3,500 | 3,500 | 3,500 |
| Total Carbohydrate (g) | 180 | 225 | 270 | 300 | 330 | 375 |
| Fiber (g) | 14 | 17 | 21 | 23* | 25 | 29* |
| Protein (g) | 30 | 38 | 45 | 50 | 55 | 63 |

*These Daily Values appear rounded up or down on food labels.

packaged foods you eat throughout the day to meet your daily goals while working toward your targets.

These are general recommendations; if you are working with a dietitian, he or she may have specific nutrient recommendations for you.

## Making choices at the grocery store

Of course, not everything at the grocery store has food labels. Vegetables, fruits, legumes, and grains—the foods that come almost directly from the earth to you—usually don't include nutrition information.

It can be difficult to remember all the guidelines and numbers when you're at the grocery store. To make it easier, first consider your targets—are you focusing on weight loss, cutting back on salt, or increasing your fiber intake? Keeping your targets in mind as you shop will help you choose foods that will support your goals—and help keep you from getting overwhelmed.

| Food Group | Typical Store Location(s) | Best Choices |
| --- | --- | --- |
| Fruits | Produce Aisle<br>Canned Goods<br>Freezer Aisle<br>Salad Bar | Variety! Fresh, frozen, canned, and dried fruits. To reduce calories and sugars, choose canned fruits packed in juice, not syrup. |
| Vegetables | Produce Aisle<br>Canned Goods<br>Freezer Aisle<br>Salad Bar<br>Pasta, Rice, and Bean Aisle | Variety! Fresh, frozen, and canned (especially dark green and orange). Dried beans and peas. To reduce sodium, look for canned vegetables packed without salt or with reduced salt. |
| Grains | Bakery<br>Bread Aisle<br>Pasta and Rice Aisle(s)<br>Cereal Aisle | Whole grains for at least half of choices. Look for whole grains as first ingredient. (See page 47 for more information on whole grains.) |
| Milk, Yogurt, and Cheese (calcium-rich foods) | Dairy Case<br>Refrigerated Aisle | Non-fat and low-fat milk and yogurt, low-fat and fat-free cheeses |
| Meat and Beans<br>Fish, Poultry, and Eggs, Soy and Nuts (protein foods) | Deli<br>Meat and Poultry Case<br>Seafood Counter<br>Egg Case<br>Canned Goods<br>Salad Bar | Lean meats, skinless poultry, fish, legumes (dried beans and peas), and nuts. |
| Oils, Condiments, and Salad Dressings | Various aisles | Monounsaturated oils like olive, canola, and peanut, and polyunsaturated oils like corn, safflower, sesame, and sunflower. Reduced calorie or low-fat salad dressings and mayonnaise. Flavored vinegars and mustards to add flavor without adding lots of fat and calories. |

Adapted from *http://www.nutrition.gov/index.php?mode=whole_story&story_id=161*

## Choosing Whole Grains

Choosing brown bread doesn't necessarily mean you're getting whole grains. To get all the benefits of whole grains, make sure the ingredients list says "whole-wheat flour," not just "wheat flour" or "enriched wheat flour." Whole-wheat flour, brown rice, rye flour, barley, or oats should be the first ingredient listed. You can also look for the Whole Grain stamp, which shows that the food provides at least 8 grams of whole grains in one serving. Breads aren't the only source of whole grains. Crackers, pastas, tortillas, cereals, and other foods can also contain whole grains; read food labels, and look for the Whole-Grain stamp to be sure.

# WEIGHT LOSS

For many people with diabetes, losing weight is one of the most important things they can do to support good health. Sometimes, losing just 5 to 10% of your weight will lower blood glucose. Work with a dietitian to create a weight-loss plan that fits your life.

The only way to lose weight is to take in fewer calories than your body uses up in a day. You can do that by eating fewer calories, burning more calories each day, or both. Most people lose more weight, and see other health benefits, by cutting calories and increasing exercise at the same time. Plus, people who do both are also more likely to keep the weight off. Either way, a slow and steady weight loss is the safest way to reach and maintain your goal.

Let's talk first about taking in fewer calories. For more information about exercise, both for weight loss and general health, see the "Exercise" section, on page 49.

## Ways to eat less

"Eating less" actually means "eating fewer calories." To do this, you may choose to eat smaller portions, or you may choose to eat the same amount of food, but eat foods that are lower in

## Tips to Eat Less

- Serve food in the kitchen. Leave the food there instead of putting it on the table. Going for seconds won't be as easy.
- Eat slowly and stop when you just begin to feel full.
- Don't watch TV, read, or listen to the radio while you eat. These activities may draw your attention away from how much you are eating and whether you are full.
- Ask another family member to put leftovers away. That way, you won't be tempted to eat the remaining food.
- Brush your teeth right after you eat. This gets the taste of food out of your mouth and may get the thought of food out of your head.
- Don't go grocery shopping when you are hungry. You may buy too much, or you may buy things that aren't on your meal plan.
- Write out a grocery list before you go shopping. Buy only what is on the list.
- Store food out of sight.
- Eat something before you go to a social function. That way, you'll be less likely to overeat fatty foods.
- Don't skip meals. You may overeat at your next one.
- Don't forbid yourself to eat certain foods, because you'll only want them more. Try to cut down on the size of the serving or the number of times you eat that food in a week. Remember, it's the first bite that tastes best. Savor it.

calories. Fat has more than twice as many calories as carbohydrate or protein. So, if you eat less fat and more carbohydrate and protein, you will take in fewer calories. The meal plan guidelines at the beginning of this chapter are a good starting point.

## Weight-loss programs

Some people may enjoy enrolling in a weight-loss program to help them lose weight. Some, like Weight Watchers and Jenny Craig, are available to anyone who wants to lose weight, not just people with diabetes. Your local hospital or medical center may also offer weight-loss classes or support groups specifically

## When Diet and Exercise Are Not Enough

Sometimes, people who are very overweight are unable to lose weight with diet and exercise alone. If you are one of these people, you may benefit from prescription weight-loss drugs or surgery. Most prescription weight-loss drugs work by making you feel less hungry. Not everyone responds the same way to weight loss drugs, and some people lose more weight than others.

Surgery may be a weight-loss option for people with type 2 diabetes if their BMI is between 35 and 40. One of the benefits of this type of weight-loss approach is that people usually experience rapid weight loss right after the surgery; however, there are risks associated with surgery that include surgical complications, gallstones, and problems absorbing nutrients.

Your health care provider can help you determine whether prescription weight-loss medication or surgery is right for you. An important thing to remember is that even if you have surgery or use weight-loss medications, it's important to change your eating habits to really be healthy.

for people with diabetes. Before you enroll in any weight-loss program, talk with your diabetes care provider. Also, when comparing programs, look for one that:

- Teaches you about nutrition and healthy food choices
- Includes regular follow-up visits for evaluation
- Encourages an increase in physical activity
- Helps you learn ways to replace old habits with new, healthier ones

# EXERCISE

Remember, the best way to lose weight is to cut calories and exercise more. Exercise is important for weight loss because it helps burn calories. It also speeds up your metabolism, which means that you'll burn more calories even when you're not exercising. Exercise may also keep you from gaining weight back once you've reached your weight-loss goal.

Even if you aren't trying to lose weight, exercise can be an important part of your diabetes care plan. Everyone with type 2 diabetes can benefit from exercise. Exercise lowers blood glucose levels and often improves the way insulin works in the body. It can help you better manage your diabetes and helps prevent common diabetes complications like circulatory and heart problems.

## Benefits of Exercise

- Prevents or delays the onset of type 2 diabetes
- Improves insulin action
- Lowers blood glucose levels
- Improves A1C in type 2 diabetes
- Lowers blood pressure and cholesterol
- Improves BMI and helps you lose weight

## Before you begin

Before you start any new exercise or exercise program, discuss your plans with your health care team. You'll want to be sure that the exercises you have planned are safe for you. Your heart, blood vessels, blood pressure, blood fat levels, and A1C levels may all be influenced by exercise; you may need to check some or all of them before you begin. Some exercises may make any heart, eye, foot, or nerve problems you have worse. Find out from your health care team what kinds of exercises are safe for you to do. Pick exercises that will work all your muscle groups (legs and hips, chest, back, shoulders, arms, and abdomen). You may want to work with an exercise physiologist or physical therapist to tailor an exercise program to your needs.

If you are new to exercise, you can introduce new habits in steps. Remember, your body is burning calories, and your muscles are working whenever you move. You can get more exercise just by changing some of the ways you do things each day. For example, whenever you drive somewhere, park your car at the far end of the parking lot and walk those extra steps to your destination. Simple changes like this can add up. (For more ideas, see "Get Moving," below.)

If you want to see how these changes add up, buy a pedometer and wear it all day. These inexpensive devices count how many steps you take while you are wearing them. They are small and clip right to your waistband or can be attached to your shoelaces. Wear one for a few weeks, and record how many steps you take each day. Try to add 500 steps every few weeks. Set a goal for yourself. Over time, try to build up to an average of 10,000 steps a day, which equals about 5 miles. Some people find they can reach 10,000 steps a day by just doing their regular daily activities and adding some of the ideas in "Get Moving," below, while most people usually

## Get Moving

If you don't exercise, you can be more active. Get on your feet and move around. When you are on your feet and moving around, you are using two to three times more energy than when you are sitting. Here are some ways to get moving:

- Get up to change TV channels instead of using the remote.
- Walk around your house during TV commercials.
- Wash dishes, load the dishwasher, or load the clothes washer or dryer during commercials.
- Use a push lawn mower rather than an electric one.
- Plant and maintain an herb or vegetable garden.
- Volunteer to work for a school or hospital.
- Walk to the subway or bus stop.
- Take the stairs rather than the elevator.
- Walk during lunch, during your break, while the oven is preheating, or while waiting for your prescription.
- If possible, walk or bike to do your errands at the local post office, library, and grocery store.
- Park your car farther away from your destination.

need to add walking to their daily activities to accomplish their goal of 10,000 steps.

## Safe exercising

Once you get moving, you may want to add some more formal exercise to your routine. That may be walking in your neighborhood each day, taking an exercise class, swimming laps at a local pool, or joining a local gym. Whatever you choose, make sure that your plan is approved by your health care team. There are three basic types of exercise: aerobic, strength, and flexibility. All three types of exercise are important to your health.

*Aerobic exercises* are ones that make your heart beat faster and make you breathe harder. Things like walking, running, riding a bike, and swimming are examples of aerobic exercise. Regular aerobic exercises can help burn extra glucose in the blood and improve the way your body uses insulin. It can also help you reach weight-loss targets by burning body fat and helping you lose weight.

*Strength exercises* are ones that work your muscles. You can do strength exercises in many ways: with weight machines, free weights, or even elastic bands. Strength exercises make your muscles stronger and your bones sturdier. Strong muscles and bones are less likely to become injured. Plus, strength exercises can also help you burn body fat and lose weight, because muscles use more calories.

*Flexibility exercises* help you stretch your muscles around your joints without stiffness or pain. Flexible muscles and joints are less likely to get injured when you use them. Everyone loses some flexibility as they get older; doing flexibility exercises regularly will help keep you active.

You'll also want to make sure that you're doing your chosen exercise correctly and safely. If you exercise incorrectly, you might injure yourself. If the exercises you have chosen require you to use equipment that is new to you, learn how to use and adjust it. Find out how to use any safety equipment that goes along with your exercise, too, such as safety goggles for racquetball and a bicycle helmet for cycling.

Each time you exercise, warm up for 5 to 10 minutes before the exercise, and cool down for 5 to 10 minutes after the exercise. A warm-up will slowly raise your heart rate, warm your muscles, and help prevent injuries. A cool-down will lower your heart rate and slow your breathing. This can be as simple as doing your exercise activity, like walking or bicycling, more slowly that normal, followed by gentle stretches.

## ADA's Recommendations for Physical Activity

ADA recommends that people with type 2 diabetes get the following amount of physical activity every week.
- At least 150 minutes of moderate-intensity aerobic activity per week.
- Resistance training at least three times per week (on nonconsecutive days).

## How long and how often to exercise

If you are just starting to exercise after a long time of little or no activity, go slowly. Doing too much too fast can lead to injuries that could keep you from doing anything at all. Plus, it's easy to get discouraged and quit when you're sore and uncomfortable. Ease into your new exercise habit to keep yourself safe and on track.

Try starting with just 5 minutes of aerobic exercise each day for 1 or 2 weeks. Then add 5 more minutes, then another 5. Gradually build up to doing 20 to 30 minutes of continuous aerobic exercise 5 times a week.

If that seems like too much time out of your schedule, consider dividing your exercise time up throughout the day.

For example, you might try brisk walking or stair climbing for 10 minutes three times a day. You'll get the same benefits, and it might be easier to stick with.

When you're ready to start strength exercises, try to do each exercise eight to 15 times. That is called a *set*. As you become stronger, you will be able to do more sets. Always rest for 30 seconds between sets to let your muscles recover. Slowly work your way up until you can do two or three sets of each exercise. Once you are doing two or three sets easily, you are ready to make the exercise harder by adding more weight. Try to do strength exercises for 20 to 30 minutes two or three times a week. Allow your muscles at least one day of rest between days you do the same strength exercises; for example, you could do arm exercises one day, and then leg exercises the next, but don't do arm exercises two days in a row.

## Signs You Are Exercising Too Hard

- You can't talk while exercising.
- Your heart rate is higher than the heart rate you are trying to maintain.
- You rate your level of exertion as hard or very hard.

## How hard to exercise

You can figure out how hard to exercise by knowing your target heart rate range. You can take your pulse by placing the tips of your first two fingers lightly over one of the blood vessels on your neck, just to the left or right of your Adam's apple. Or try the pulse spot inside your wrist just below the base of your thumb. (Caution: Do not check your pulse on both sides of your neck at the same time. You may interrupt blood flow to the brain enough to cause loss of consciousness and possibly a stroke.) Count your pulse for 6 seconds and then add a 0 to the end. For example, if you counted 8 heartbeats in

6 seconds, then your beats per minute equal 80. Your health care provider can help you decide the target heart rate that is best for you. The basic formula for figuring out your target heart rate is below.

## Finding Your Target Heart Rate

220 – your age = your maximum heart rate in beats per minute.
× 0.60 = your minimum working heart rate in beats per minute.
× 0.80 = your maximum working heart rate in beats per minute.

Using this formula, if you are 55 years old:
220 – 55 = 165 beats per minute.
165 × 0.60 = 99 beats per minute.
165 × 0.80 = 132 beats per minute.

This means your target heart-rate range during exercise is between 99 beats per minute (60% of your maximum heart rate) and 132 beats per minute (80% of your maximum heart rate).

You can compare this to your working heart rate range to see whether you are on target. If you have nerve damage or take certain blood pressure drugs, your heart may beat more slowly. If your heart does beat more slowly, your heart rate is not a good guide for how hard to exercise. Instead, exercise at what you feel is a moderate level of exertion. You should be able to talk while you're exercising, and you should not feel that you are working too hard.

## When and what to drink

Exercise makes you sweat. Sweating means you are losing fluid. To replace lost fluids, be sure to drink before and after exercise or, if the exercise is intense, during exercise.

Water is usually the best choice. But if you are exercising for a long time, you may want a drink that contains carbohydrate. Choose drinks that are no more than 10% carbohydrate, such as sports drinks or diluted fruit juices (1/2 cup fruit juice plus 1/2 cup water).

## When to exercise

A good time to exercise is 1 to 3 hours after you finish a meal or snack. The food you have eaten will help keep your blood glucose level from falling too low.

## When not to exercise

Do not exercise when:

- You are dehydrated
- You are short of breath
- You are ill
- You have a serious injury
- You feel dizzy
- You feel sick to your stomach
- You have pain/tightness in your chest, neck, shoulders, or jaw
- You have blurred sight or blind spots

## When to Check Your Blood Glucose

As we've explained, exercise can affect your blood glucose levels. Most of the time, exercise causes blood glucose levels to go down—usually a good thing for people with diabetes.

But if you take insulin or some types of diabetes pills, exercise can cause your blood glucose level to go too low. If you take insulin or diabetes pills, the only way to know how exercise will affect you is to check your blood glucose before and after exercising. After a few times, you'll get an idea of how your blood glucose levels are affected by exercise and, if needed, you can make changes to your medication, eating plan, or exercise schedule. You may want to talk with your health care team about the effects you see and the best way to manage them.

## How to stick with it

- *Convenience.* Choose a type of exercise you can do with a minimum of travel time and preparation. Find something that you can fit easily into your daily routine. Some people find walking at lunchtime convenient. For others, riding a stationary bike at home or taking an exercise class close to home works better.
- *Cost.* Select an activity that requires a minimum of special equipment, clothes, or fees. Consider secondhand exercise equipment. Check out exercise classes at community recreation centers, churches, and schools, where prices are usually reasonable.
- *Classes.* Many communities offer a variety of exercise classes. Be cautious, however. Not all exercise classes are of equal quality. Watch or try out at least one class before signing up. Look for instructors who are certified and have training in CPR (cardiopulmonary resuscitation). You might also want to ask whether the instructor has experience teaching people with diabetes. Be sure classes include a warm-up, heart-rate monitoring, and a cooldown that includes stretching.
- *Goals.* Set realistic and measurable goals. Break down the goals so you can see your progress. For example, if you're starting a walking program, a short-term goal might be walking for 10 minutes three times a week.
- *Rewards.* When you reach a goal, give yourself a reward, such as a new CD, book, or article of clothing.
- *Enjoyment.* Find activities that you enjoy. If you're the social type, chances are you'll enjoy an exercise class. If you value time alone, perhaps swimming laps is for you.
- *Support.* Find someone to exercise with; ask a friend or relative to take a class with you. Making the commitment to meet someone for exercise can help get you out the door.

- *Learning.* Read up on activities you enjoy. Articles, books, or personal accounts of others who enjoy the same activity can be inspirational.
- *Novelty.* If you're bored with the same old exercise routine, try something new.

# SKIN CARE

People with diabetes are more likely to get skin infections caused by bacteria or fungus. That's because high blood glucose levels make the body's natural defenses less effective. Plus, some of the bacteria and fungi that cause infections feed off of glucose. Diabetes also causes you to pass more urine, which can lead to dry, itchy, dehydrated skin. For all of these reasons, people with diabetes need to pay extra attention to their skin and treat any skin problems quickly.

## Bacterial infections

Styes, boils, and carbuncles are three of the most common bacterial infections seen in people with diabetes. All three are caused by staphylococcal bacteria, and appear as red, painful, pus-filled lumps. Anyone can get styes, boils, and carbuncles, but they develop more easily in people with diabetes.

A stye is an infected gland of the eyelid. A boil is an infected hair root or skin gland. A carbuncle is a cluster of boils. Boils and carbuncles often occur at the back of your neck, armpits, groin, or buttocks. If you think you have a stye, boil, carbuncle, or other bacterial infection, consult your diabetes care provider.

## Fungal infections

Again, anyone can develop a fungal infection, but people with diabetes get them more easily. Most fungi like warm, moist, dark places, so fungal infections often develop in the groin area and the feet.

Men can develop **jock itch,** a red, itchy infection that spreads from the genitals outward over the inside of the thigh. Women can develop **vaginal infections,** caused by the fungus *Candida albicans.* This causes a thick, white discharge from the vagina along with itching, burning, and irritation. Both men and women can develop **athlete's foot,** a fungal infection of the feet. Athlete's foot causes the skin between your toes to become itchy and sore; the skin may also crack and peel or blister.

People with diabetes may also be more likely to get ringworm, though this type of infection is less common. Ringworm is a ring-shaped, red, scaly patch that may itch or blister. It can appear on the feet, groin, scalp, nails, or body.

If you develop one of these fungal infections, try an over-the-counter antifungal medicine first. It's a good idea to tell your diabetes care provider about any food problems you have. (See "Foot Care," page 60). If the infection doesn't get better after a few days of over-the-counter treatment, contact your diabetes care provider.

## How to Care for Your Skin

- **Keep your blood glucose in target range most of the time.** High blood glucose levels make it easier for bacteria and fungal infections to occur.
- **Keep your skin clean.** Take warm, not hot, baths or showers. Hot water can dry out your skin.
- **Keep dry skin moist.** Use moisturizers and moisturizing soaps. Keep your home more humid during cold, dry months. Drink plenty of water. It helps keep your skin moist, too.
- **Keep other parts of your skin dry.** Areas where skin touches skin need to be kept dry. These areas are between your toes, under your arms, and at your groin. Using powder on these areas can help keep them dry.
- **Protect your skin from the sun.** The sun can dry and burn your skin. When you are out in the sun, wear a waterproof, sweat-proof sunscreen with an SPF (sun protection factor) of at least 15. Wearing a hat also helps.
- **Treat minor skin problems.** Over-the-counter products can be used to treat minor skin problems. Check with your doctor before using any products.
- **See a skin doctor.** If you are prone to skin problems, ask your diabetes care provider for a referral to a skin doctor (dermatologist).

# FOOT CARE

People with diabetes are prone to foot problems, for many of the same reasons that they are prone to skin problems. High blood glucose levels weaken the body's natural defenses against infection and dry out the skin. Diabetes can also cause nerve damage that makes it harder to feel pain in the feet. Because even minor problems can quickly become serious for people with diabetes, caring for your feet is an important part of your care plan.

## Corns and calluses

Calluses are areas of thick skin caused by regular or prolonged pressure or friction. A corn is a callus on a toe. Corns and calluses can develop on your feet when your body weight is borne unevenly, or when you wear shoes that rub or are too tight. There are several things you can do to prevent calluses from forming:

*Wear shoes that fit.* Shoes that fit are comfortable when you buy them. Almost all new shoes are a little stiff at the start and mold to your feet with wear, but this is different from buying shoes and trying to break them in. Make sure there is room for you to move your toes.

*Wear shoes with low heels and thick soles.* Thick soles will cushion and protect your feet. Low heels distribute your weight more evenly.

*Try padded socks.* They not only cushion and protect feet but also reduce pressure. Be sure your shoe is large enough to fit this thicker sock. You may need extra-deep shoes.

*Try shoe inserts.* Ask your diabetes care provider or foot doctor about shoe inserts to better distribute your weight.

If you get a callus or corn, don't try to deal with it yourself—see your diabetes care provider or foot doctor. Trying to trim or cut it yourself can lead to an infection, and over-the-counter medicines can burn your skin. Be sure to see a professional as soon as possible—untrimmed calluses can get very thick, break down, and turn into ulcers, a much more serious problem.

## Foot ulcers

Foot ulcers are open sores or holes in the skin. Ulcers can be caused by an untreated cut, callus, or blister, most often on the ball of the foot or the bottom of the big toe. They can also develop on the sides of the foot, usually due to shoes that don't fit well. You can prevent ulcers by:

- Wearing shoes that fit
- Wearing new shoes for just a few hours at a time
- Throwing away worn-out shoes and sneakers
- Wearing socks that fit
- Wearing socks without holes, or bumpy areas in them
- Checking for pebbles or other objects before you put on your shoes

An ulcer can be very painful; however, if you have nerve damage (see page 62), you may not feel it. Even though you may not feel any pain from an ulcer, you need to see your diabetes care provider or podiatrist (foot doctor) right away. Walking on an ulcer can cause it to become larger and infected. If not treated, an infected ulcer can lead to gangrene and amputation. (See Chapter 5 for more information about these complications.)

## Poor circulation

Poor circulation causes your feet to feel cold and look blue or swollen. The best way to treat cold feet is to wear warm socks, even to bed. Do not use hot water bottles, heating pads, or electric blankets—they may burn your feet without you noticing. Test bathwater first with your elbow to avoid burning your feet. If your feet are often swollen, try lace-up shoes. You can tighten or loosen them as needed.

To increase blood flow to your feet, try exercise (with your health provider's approval). Smoking also limits blood flow to your feet; if you smoke and want to stop, ask your diabetes care provider for advice on quitting.

## Nerve damage (neuropathy)

Nerve damage causes your feet to become numb, so you are less able to feel pain, heat, and cold. If you have lost some feeling, you could hurt your foot and not notice. People with nerve damage need to take special steps to protect their feet. If you are going swimming or wading, wear footwear made for water. Also, check your shoes before you put them on. Make sure there are no stones, nails, paper clips, pins, or other sharp objects in them. Be sure the inside of the shoe is smooth and free of tears or rough edges.

Nerve damage can also affect the nerves that cause sweating. As a result, your feet may become dry and scaly, and the skin may peel and crack. Soaking your feet will also dry out your skin. If your feet have become dry and scaly, you can rub lotion on them as needed; however, avoid putting lotion between your toes, because the extra moisture there can lead to infection.

Nerve damage can cause your feet to become misshapen. Your toes may curl up, the ball of your foot may stick out more, and your arch may get higher. These changes can cause some parts of your feet to bear more weight. Those areas are then more likely to get calluses and corns. If the shape of your feet has changed, ask your diabetes care provider or foot doctor about shoe inserts or special shoes.

## How to Care for Your Feet

- **Check both your feet each day.** Look all over them. Compare one foot to the other. Look for cuts, blisters, scratches, ingrown toenails, changes in color, changes in shape, punctures, or anything that wasn't there the day before. If you cannot see well, have a friend or relative check your feet for you, or use a mirror to see the bottoms of your feet.
- **Keep your toenails trimmed.** Trim your toenails to follow the curve of your toe. If you can't trim them yourself, your podiatrist can do it for you.
- **Have your feet checked regularly.** Take your shoes and socks off at every regular office visit to remind your health care provider to check your feet. Remind your diabetes care provider to check your feet for blood vessel, muscle, and nerve damage at least once a year.
- **Keep your diabetes care provider informed.** Call your provider if you have a sore on your foot that won't heal, or any other foot problem, no matter how minor.

# DENTAL CARE

Having diabetes puts you at risk for gum disease and other mouth infections because high levels of glucose in the blood make the body's natural defenses less effective. Plus, some of the bacteria that cause infections feed off of glucose. You can protect yourself by knowing the signs of gum disease and other mouth infections, and by knowing how to take care of your teeth.

## Gum disease

Gum disease starts when a sticky film of bacteria, called *plaque*, forms on your teeth and at your gum line. Brushing and flossing your teeth removes the plaque. If plaque is not removed, it hardens into tartar. Plaque and tartar can make your gums red, sore, and swollen and cause them to bleed when you brush or floss. This is called *gingivitis*.

If gingivitis is not treated, your gums may begin to pull away from your teeth. Pockets may form between your teeth and gums and fill with bacteria and pus. This is called *periodontitis*. Periodontitis can destroy bone. Your teeth may start to move. You may notice a change in the way your teeth fit when you bite or in the way your partial dentures fit. Your teeth may get loose, fall out, or have to be pulled.

## Other mouth infections

Mouth infections affect small areas in your mouth rather than your whole mouth. They can be caused by bacteria or a fungus. Know the warning signs of mouth infections:

- Swelling around your teeth or gums or anywhere in your mouth
- Pus around your teeth or gums or anywhere in your mouth
- White or red patches anywhere in your mouth
- Pain in your mouth or sinuses that does not go away
- Dark spots or holes on your teeth
- Teeth that hurt when you eat something cold, hot, or sweet
- Pain when chewing

## How to protect your teeth

### Keep your blood glucose on target
If you keep your blood glucose close to target range, you'll lower your risk of gum disease and other mouth infections.

### Keep your teeth clean
Flossing or using dental picks cleans plaque and bits of food from between your teeth. Brushing removes plaque and bits of food from the surfaces of your teeth. Brush your teeth with a fluoride toothpaste, and floss at least twice a day. Better yet, brush and floss after every meal. A soft toothbrush with

## Tips for Daily Dental Care

1. Place the toothbrush at a 45-degree angle to where the teeth meet the gums.
2. Gently move the brush back and forth in short strokes on the outer tooth surfaces.
3. Brush the inner tooth surfaces. Use the tip of the brush for the inner front tooth surfaces. Brush the chewing surfaces. Brush the upper surface of your tongue.
4. Break off about 18 inches of floss, and wind most of it around one of your middle fingers.
5. Wind the remaining floss around the same finger of the other hand. This finger will take up the floss as it is used.
6. Hold the floss tightly between your thumb and forefingers, with about 1 inch of floss between them. Use a gentle "sawing motion" to guide the floss between your teeth.
7. When the floss reaches the gum line, curve it into a C-shape against one tooth. Gently slide it into the space between the gum and the tooth until you feel resistance. Hold the floss against the tooth. Gently scrape the side of the tooth, moving the floss away from the gum.

rounded or polished bristles is easiest on your gums. Be sure to replace your toothbrush every 3 or 4 months, or sooner if the bristles are worn.

### See your dentist

Have your dentist or dental hygienist clean your teeth at least every 6 months. These cleanings get rid of plaque and tartar. Make sure your dentist takes complete mouth X-rays every 2 years to check for bone loss. For some people, bone loss is the only sign of periodontitis. Consult your dentist if you have any of the signs of gum disease or other mouth infections.

# SICK DAYS

It's easy for your blood glucose levels to get out of control when you are sick. Your illness may make you lose your appetite, making it difficult to follow your meal plan. Even if you are able to eat as you usually do, your blood glucose level will probably be higher than usual. Your body reacts to sickness by releasing certain hormones that can make blood glucose go up.

It's important for people with diabetes to have a sick-day plan. Ask your health care team to help you make a sick-day plan before you get sick. Your sick-day plan will include how often to test your blood glucose, how to manage your medicines, what to eat and drink, when to call your diabetes care provider, and what to tell him or her.

Even if you usually only check your blood glucose once a day, you'll probably want to check more often when you are sick. As explained above, when you're sick, your body releases hormones that can make blood glucose go up. Ask your diabetes care team about how often you should check when you are sick. As a starting point, you may need to check every 3 or 4 hours.

## Managing medicines

If you take insulin and/or diabetes pills, it's important to continue taking them when you're sick. Remember, your blood

### When to Call Your Provider

Call your health care provider if:

- You have been sick for one or two days, and you are not getting better
- You have been vomiting or have had diarrhea for more than 6 hours
- You are taking diabetes pills, and your pre-meal blood glucose levels are 250 mg/dl or higher for more than 24 hours
- You are taking insulin, and your blood glucose level is staying above 250 mg/dl or the target set by you and your provider
- You have any of these signs: very dry mouth, fruity breath, dry and cracked lips or tongue, stomach pain, chest pain, difficulty breathing, confusion, or disorientation
- You are sleepier than normal
- You are not sure what to do to take care of yourself

glucose tends to go up when you are sick, even if you are not eating.

You may need other kinds of medicines to care for your sickness. Some of these medicines, particularly cough and cold remedies, may have ingredients in them that can raise your blood glucose level. Also, some contain sugar and alcohol. Read labels carefully for active ingredients and inactive ingredients. Look for sugar-free and alcohol-free versions of the same medicine. Ask your pharmacist or diabetes care provider whether the medicines you plan to take will affect your blood glucose level. (See Chapter 5 for a list of medicines that can affect blood glucose.)

For headache and fever, aspirin should be fine; however, people with diabetes should avoid ibuprofen, the medicine in brands like Advil and Motrin. If you have kidney disease, check with your doctor first before taking it, because ibuprofen is not safe for people with kidney disease.

## What About Flu Shots and Pneumonia Shots?

People with diabetes are four times as likely to die from the flu or pneumonia as people without diabetes. It is recommended that most people with diabetes get a flu shot once a year. The shot makes it harder to catch the flu, and even if you do catch the flu, your symptoms will likely be milder. If you are allergic to eggs, do not get a flu shot. Pneumonia shots are also recommended for many people with diabetes. Medicare and most insurers will cover the costs for these shots.

## What to eat and drink

Follow your usual meal plan if you can. If you can't eat your usual foods, use your sick-day meal plan. It should include foods that are easy on your stomach and appeal to you when you are sick. You may want to set aside a small area of your cupboard for foods on your sick-day plan so you will be prepared.

## Sick-Day Foods and Fluids with Close to 15g Carbohydrate per Serving

Here are some ideas for sick-day foods and drinks. Check labels as brands will vary. Work with your dietitian to choose a sick-day meal plan that appeals to you.

- Regular ice cream (1/2 cup)—15 grams
- Low-fat ice cream (1/2 cup)—10 grams
- Fruit juice bar (3 ounces)—9 grams
- Frozen yogurt (1/2 cup)—15 grams
- Gelatin or Jello sweetened (1/2 cup)—19 grams
- Toast (1 slice)—15 grams
- Soup (1 cup)—15 grams
- Chicken noodle soup (1 cup)—9 grams
- Cream soup (1 cup)—9 grams (made with water)
- Tomato soup (1 cup)—16 grams (made with water)
- Applesauce, unsweetened (1/2 cup)—14 grams
- Apple juice (1/2 cup)—15 grams
- Grape juice (1/3 cup)—12 grams
- Ginger ale (1/2 cup)—10 grams
- Sports drink (1 cup)—14 grams
- Regular cola or root beer (1/2 cup)—14 grams

If you have a fever, are vomiting, or have diarrhea, you may lose a lot of fluid. Try to drink 3 to 6 ounces of fluid each hour by taking a few sips every few minutes. Non-diet, decaffeinated soft drinks or sports drinks with sugar and carbohydrate can help prevent *hypoglycemia* (low blood glucose).

### How About Exercise When I'm Sick?

Exercising when you are sick can make your blood glucose levels go down too low or up too high. If you exercise when you are sick, it may take longer for you to get better. Find out from your health care provider when it is safe to start exercising again. Because you may be less fit after being sick, ease into your exercise program. You might try exercising at a lower intensity, for a shorter time, or on fewer days.

# PREGNANCY

Diabetes can impact many areas of your health. That's true of pregnancy as well. Women with diabetes can have healthy pregnancies and healthy babies; however, it is even more important for women with diabetes to keep their blood glucose level close to normal before and during pregnancy. High blood glucose levels put your baby at higher risk for certain health problems, such as becoming very large; having difficulty breathing; low blood glucose; or *jaundice*, a yellowing of the skin. Although most of these conditions can be treated, preventing them in the first place is better for your baby.

## How to Ensure Your Baby's Health

- **Plan your pregnancy.** Stay on birth control until your blood glucose is at target. This is important because high glucose levels and some diabetes medications can cause birth defects.
- **Keep your blood glucose in the target range for pregnancy.** You will need to manage your blood glucose intensively, which will include more frequent monitoring.
- **Get fit before you get pregnant.** Exercising before pregnancy may increase your endurance, help lower your blood glucose, help you lose weight, and build strength and flexibility.
- **Exercise during your pregnancy.** Pregnancy is not the time to start a vigorous exercise program, but you will most likely be able to continue any exercise you were doing regularly before pregnancy. If you were not exercising regularly, ask your obstetrician about exercises that would be safe for you and your baby.
- **Use your meal plan.** A pregnancy meal plan is not designed to help you lose weight—it is to help you avoid high and low blood glucose while providing what your baby needs to grow. Your plan will likely change during your pregnancy to keep up with your body's and the baby's needs.

## Questions you may have about your pregnancy:

### Should I still take my diabetes pills?

No. Diabetes pills are not used during pregnancy. Insulin will be used to manage your blood glucose levels before conception and during pregnancy.

### If I already take insulin, will my dose change?

Most likely. You may need two or three times more insulin during pregnancy, especially toward the end of pregnancy.

### What about alcohol, drugs, and other medications?

Many medications can be harmful to your baby. Check with your health care provider before taking any prescription or over-the-counter medications.

Avoid drinking alcohol when you are pregnant and even when you are trying to conceive. Don't smoke cigarettes or use illegal drugs when pregnant. All of these may seriously harm your baby.

### Is it OK to breastfeed?

Yes. Breastfeeding can be a wonderful experience for you and your baby. Breast milk gives your baby *antibodies* (protection against infection) and allergy-proof nutrition that no canned formula can duplicate.

You will probably find yourself hungrier and thirstier while breastfeeding. Therefore, you'll need a meal plan designed to give you and your baby the nutrients you both need.

Breastfeeding may affect your blood glucose levels. You may find you have erratic blood glucose levels and more low blood glucose levels. On the other hand, you may find your glucose is easier to manage, and you may be able to eat a little more and take less medication. Your medications will need to be adjusted for breastfeeding and again when you stop breastfeeding.

# CHAPTER 4

# Medications and Monitoring

Meal planning and exercise are usually the first steps people take in learning to manage their type 2 diabetes. Over time, many people will add diabetes pills to their care plan. Some people with type 2 diabetes will also add insulin. Diabetes is a progressive disease, so care plans often change over time to adjust to the new ways the disease is affecting your body.

## DIABETES PILLS

Diabetes pills generally work best for people who have had type 2 diabetes for less than 10 years. You may consider diabetes pills when:

- Your A1C is over 7%
- Your blood glucose levels are over 130 mg/dl before a meal
- Your blood glucose levels are over 180 mg/dl after a meal

There are five different classes of diabetes pills prescribed in the United States: sulfonylureas, biguanides, thiazolidinediones, meglitinides, and alpha-glucosidase inhibitors.

## Sulfonylureas

Many diabetes pills belong to the class of drugs called sulfonyl-ureas. There are six different sulfonylureas available in the United States (See table below).

Sulfonylureas help your body send out more of its own insulin, and help your body respond to it. They also stop your liver from putting stored glucose into your blood. These actions lower your blood glucose. Sometimes, sulfonylureas make your blood glucose go too low—for example, if you skip meals or drink too much alcohol. You may also gain weight when you take them.

Possible side effects of sulfonylureas include nausea, vomiting, a skin rash, and itching. Tell your diabetes care provider about any side effects you notice. Do not take sulfonyl-ureas if you are pregnant, have allergies to sulfa drugs, or have severe liver or kidney disease.

### Sulfonylureas

| Generic Name | Brand Name | Action Time | Doses per Day |
|---|---|---|---|
| Glipizide | Glucotrol<br>Glucotrol XL | Intermediate<br>Long | 1 or 2 |
| Glimepiride | Amaryl | Long | 1 |
| Glyburide | Diabeta<br>Micronase<br>Glynase PresTab | Intermediate | 1 or 2 |

## Biguanides

Biguanide metformin (brand name Glucophage) is an intermediate-acting pill that is taken two or three times a day. Metformin causes your liver to release stored glucose more slowly. It may also help your body respond to insulin. Metformin helps lower your fasting blood glucose levels—the levels seen before you eat. It does not help your body send out more insulin, so there is very little chance of low blood glucose and weight gain.

Possible side effects of metformin include a metallic taste in your mouth, an upset stomach, nausea, loss of appetite, and diarrhea. These side effects usually go away after a time. If you have heart, kidney, or liver disease, do not take metformin, because it can cause you to develop lactic acidosis—a life-threatening build-up of acid in the blood.

## Thiazolidinediones

The thiazolidinediones rosiglitazone (brand name Avandia) and pioglitazone (brand name Actos) are approved for use in people with type 2 diabetes who are taking insulin. Thiazolidinediones enhance the action of insulin so that your body needs less. They have also been shown to lower triglyceride levels and raise HDL (the good) cholesterol levels. Because they may cause fluid retention, these drugs are not recommended for people with congestive heart disease. They have also been linked to bone fractures. Rosiglitazone has been associated with an increased risk of heart attack.

## Meglitinides

Meglitinide repaglinide (brand name Prandin) and meglitinide natiglinide (brand name Starlix) are usually prescribed for people whose type 2 diabetes can't be controlled by diet and exercise alone. Meglitinides differ from other diabetes pills in that they work very quickly and are taken just prior to eating—anytime from 30 minutes before meals to right before you eat. They work by helping your pancreas release more insulin during and just after a meal. This results in smaller meal-related increases in blood glucose. Because repaglinides are eliminated from the bloodstream within 3 to 4 hours, it does not cause your body to release insulin over long periods of time.

Side effects of repaglinide are rare but may include low blood glucose, upper respiratory infections, nausea, diarrhea, constipation, joint pain, and headache.

## Alpha-glucosidase inhibitors

The alpha-glucosidase inhibitors acarbose (brand name Precose) and miglitol (brand name Glyset) are pills taken three times a day, with main meals. These drugs work by slowing the time it takes for your intestines to break food down into glucose. This causes glucose to enter your blood more slowly. Acarbose and miglitol may be helpful at flattening out the sharp rise in glucose that may occur after meals.

Possible side effects of alpha-glucosidase inhibitors include gas, bloating, and diarrhea. Most people get these side effects when they first begin using the drugs, then after a while the side effects go away; however, some people will still have them. Do not take acarbose or miglitol if you have any gastrointestinal diseases.

You and your diabetes care provider will need to work together to find the best treatment. It will be important for you to keep records of when you take your medication and the dosage. It will help to check your blood glucose more often until you find the right doses for you.

# OTHER MEDICATIONS

You may take other prescription or over-the-counter medications. It's important to know how these medications act inside your body and how they interact with each other. Some medications may lower or raise your blood glucose level or interfere with how your body uses diabetes pills (See box on next page).

# Medications That Can Affect Blood Glucose Levels

| Generic Name | Brand Name | Effect on Blood Glucose Level | Interacts with Diabetes Pills? | Common Uses |
|---|---|---|---|---|
| Alcohol | Ingredient in many medications | Lowers | Yes | Carry active ingredient in drug into metabolism |
| Aspirin | Many brand names | May lower if taken in large doses | Yes | Treat general pain or fever; treat arthritis; and may prevent heart attack (low doses taken for prevention of heart attack) Do not affect blood glucose |
| Beta-blockers | Inderal Sectral Tenormin Lopressor Visken Blocadren | May mask low blood glucose | Yes | Treat high blood pressure, angina, irregular heartbeat, overactive thyroid, and other ailments |
| Chloramphenicol | Chloromycetin | Lowers* | Yes | Treat bacterial infections |
| Clofibrate | Atromid-S | Lowers* | Yes | Treat high cholesterol and triglyceride levels |
| Diazoxide | Hyperstat Proglycem | Raises | Yes | Treat low blood glucose caused by tumors in pancreas; sometimes used to treat high blood pressure |
| Diuretics | Diuril HydroDIURIL Edecrin Esidrix Diamox Lasix Hygroton | May raise if taken in high doses | Yes | Relieve fluid buildup by increasing amount of water in urine |
| Epinephrine | Epinephrine | Raises | Yes | Revive heartbeat; treat severe allergic reactions |

*(continued)*

## Medications That Can Affect Blood Glucose Levels *(Continued)*

| Generic Name | Brand Name | Effect on Blood Glucose Level | Interacts with Diabetes Pills? | Common Uses |
|---|---|---|---|---|
| Epinephrine-like drugs (ephedrine, pseudoephedrine phenylephrine) | Many cold, flu, and allergy medicines | Raises | Yes | Treat runny noses, flu, allergies, and colds |
| Estrogens, birth control pills | Many brand names | May raise | No | Prevent pregnancy; lessen the effects of menopause |
| Lithium carbonate | Eskalith Lithonate | Raises | No | Treat manic depression |
| Methyldopa | Aldomet | Lowers* | Yes | Treat high blood pressure |
| Monoamine oxidase (MAO) inhibitors | Parnate Nardil | Lowers | Yes | Treat severe depression |
| Nicotinic acid, niacin | Nicolar Nicobid | Raises in high doses | No | Treat nutrient deficiency; treat high cholesterol levels |
| Phenobarbital | Many brand names | Raises* | Yes | Sedate; treat epilepsy |
| Phentermine | Several brand names | Raises | Yes | Suppress appetite |
| Phenylbutazone | Butazolidin | Lowers* | Yes | Treat arthritis |
| Phenylpropanolamine | Acutrim Dexatrim | Raises | Yes | Suppress appetite |
| Phenytoin | Dilantin | Raises | Yes | Treat epilepsy and other nervous system disorders |
| Rifampin | Rifadin | Raises* | Yes | Treat tuberculosis |
| Steroids (prednisone, cortisone, dexamethasone) | Steraspred Deltasone Cortone Decadron | Raises | Yes | Reduce inflammation, redness, and swelling |
| Sulfa drugs | Gantrisin Septra Bactrim | Lowers* | Yes | Treat bacterial infections |
| Thyroid preparations | Armour S-P-T | May raise in high doses | No | Treat lessened or absent thyroid function |

*These drugs raise or lower blood glucose only when used in combination with diabetes pills.

Be sure to follow all instructions for taking your medications. Make sure all members of your health care team know what medications you are taking. Try to use a single pharmacy for all your prescriptions. That way, all your medications can be listed on one record. Check your blood glucose to see whether a new medication affects your blood glucose level. If you find that a medication you are taking greatly upsets your blood glucose levels, ask your diabetes care provider or pharmacist about it.

# INSULIN

Many people think of diabetes as a sugar problem, but remember, diabetes is really a problem with insulin. In type 2 diabetes, your body doesn't make enough insulin, or your body has a hard time using the insulin, or both. So, sometimes people with type 2 diabetes need to take extra insulin.

There are several different sources of insulin. *Human insulin* is made by putting the human gene for insulin into bacteria, causing the bacteria to make human insulin. The insulin is then extracted and purified. *Analog insulin* is created when scientists make changes to human insulin genes in a laboratory. These changes make analog insulin work more quickly and make it easier for your body to use.

## Insulin types

Aside from the source, there are also several different types of insulin. Each type works differently in the body. Insulin's action has three parts: *onset, peak time,* and *duration.* Onset is how long insulin takes to start working. Peak time is when insulin is working its hardest. Duration is how long insulin keeps working.

Some of the times for onset, peak, and duration are given as ranges in the table below. That's because insulin may work

## Insulin action

| Type of Insulin | Onset | Peak | Duration | Types |
|---|---|---|---|---|
| Rapid-acting | 15 minutes | 60 minutes | 4–5 hours | Lispro, aspart, glulisine |
| Short-acting | 30–45 minutes | 2–3 hours | 6 hours | Regular |
| Intermediate-acting | 2–4 hours | 4–10 hours | 10–16 hours | NPH |
| Very long-acting | 1 hour | – | 24 hours | Glargine, Detemir |

slower or faster in you than in someone else, and some types of insulin may work faster than others.

## Insulin mixtures

Some types of insulin combine two different types, to give you the benefits of both. This type of insulin is called *pre-mixed insulin* or *mixed insulin*. For example, an insulin mixture may combine intermediate-acting insulin with a smaller portion of short-acting insulin. The chart below includes information on the most common insulin mixtures.

Some people make their own insulin mixtures, by combining two types of insulin in one syringe. But now that you can buy pre-mixed insulin, this is less common.

## Insulin Mixtures

| | Ingredients | Types |
|---|---|---|
| 50/50 insulin | 50% intermediate-acting insulin; 50% short-acting | |
| 70/30 insulin | 70% intermediate-acting; 30% short-acting or rapid-acting | Humulin 70/30, Novolin 70/30, NovoLog Mix 70/30 |
| 75/25 insulin | 75% intermediate acting; 25% rapid acting | Humalog Mix |

## Insulin strengths

Insulin comes in different strengths. The most common strength of insulin used in the United States is U-100 insulin. This means that there are 100 units of insulin per milliliter of fluid. U-500 insulin is also available in the United States. If you inject insulin, the syringe must match the strength of your insulin.

## Insulin storage and safety

Insulin makers say you should store your unopened insulin in the refrigerator. Do not put your insulin in the freezer or allow it to warm in the sun or in a hot car. Freezing and extreme heat can destroy the potency of insulin. The vial of insulin you are using can be left at room temperature for up to a month.

Check the expiration date before opening your insulin. If the date has passed, don't use the insulin. If the date is yet to come, look closely at the insulin in the vial. Rapid-acting, short-acting, and very long-acting insulin should be clear, with no floating pieces or color. Intermediate-acting insulin and insulin mixtures should be cloudy, but without floating pieces or crystals. If the insulin does not look as it should, return the unopened vial of insulin to the place you bought it for an exchange or refund.

## Insulin injections

Insulin needs to be injected just under the skin, into the fat, to work well. One way to take insulin is by using syringes. You may have to try several brands of syringes before you find one that suits you. Pick a syringe that is:

- Large enough to hold your entire dose for each injection. For example, if you take 45 units, you cannot use a 30-unit syringe.

- Easy to read. The markings on the syringe may be easier to read if the plunger is a different color.
- Comfortable. Today's syringes have tiny, thin needles with a slick coating so they go in easily.

## Insulin Injection Tips

- Inject insulin at room temperature. Using cold insulin right from the refrigerator may make it hurt more.
- Relax your muscles in the area.
- Puncture the skin quickly.
- Keep the needle going in the same direction when you put it in and take it out.
- Use sharp needles.

## Insulin pens

You may choose to use an insulin pen instead of a syringe. It's called an insulin pen because it looks like a fountain pen. But these "pens" hold insulin instead of ink, and under the cap there is a small needle. A small dial lets you adjust the dose of insulin you get from the pen. There are reusable insulin pens, which allow you to replace used insulin cartridges with new, full ones. There are also disposable insulin pens that can be thrown away after one use. You may find that insulin pens are a convenient way to get your insulin doses when you are away from home.

## Where to inject insulin

Insulin works best when it is injected into a layer of fat under the skin. Here are several areas of the body that generally work well for insulin injection:

1. Abdomen (anywhere except within two inches of your navel or bellybutton)

2. Upper arms (outside part)
3. Buttocks (anywhere)

Insulin is absorbed at different speeds at each site. For most kinds of insulin, the fastest absorption comes from injections in the abdomen. You may prefer to inject insulin in the same area so that you know how it will act, or you may want to choose your area according to how fast or slow you want the insulin to start working. Either way, keep track of how your body responds by testing your blood glucose and recording the results.

To prevent skin problems, it is important to change the injection site every day, even if you are injecting into the same area. This is called *site rotation*. For example, you may always inject your daily dose of insulin into your abdomen, but each day you would put the needle in a different site on your abdomen.

It may help to think of each site as a circle on that area of your body. The circles, or injection sites, should be one inch

## How to Inject Insulin

1. Wash your hands with soap and water.
2. Choose an injection site. (See "Where to Inject Insulin," page 80–81.) Make sure the site is clean and dry.
3. Gently pinch a fold of skin between your thumb and forefinger.
4. Push the needle straight through the skin at a 90-degree angle. If you are thin, you may need to push the needle in at a 45-degree angle to avoid muscle.
5. Relax the pinch, and push in the plunger to inject the insulin. Keep the needle in your skin for 5–10 seconds.
6. Pull the needle straight out.
7. Cover the injection site with your finger or a dry cotton ball or gauze and apply slight pressure to the site for 5 to 8 seconds without rubbing. Rubbing may disperse the insulin too quickly or cause irritation.
8. Write down how much insulin you injected and the time of day.

apart. The number of sites you have in one area depends on how big your body is. The bigger your body, the more sites you have in each area. To rotate sites, you use a different circle for each injection until all the circles have been used up. Then you start all over again.

## How to dispose of syringes

Used syringes are considered medical waste because they have come in contact with human blood. It is important that they are disposed of properly, so that no one who handles your trash is harmed.

Check with your local health department to see if your town has special rules about the disposal of medical waste. The health department may be able to offer advice on how to dispose of your used syringes while following local laws.

The best way to dispose of syringes and needles is to place them in a puncture-proof container with a tight-fitting lid before putting them in the garbage. Heavy-duty plastic or metal containers are good choices. You don't need to buy a special container—an empty liquid laundry detergent bottle works fine. Remove the needles from the syringes before putting them in the container, to prevent anyone from reusing them.

When traveling, if possible, bring your used syringes home. You can pack them in a heavy-duty container, such as a hard plastic pencil box, for transport.

## Injection aids

Injecting insulin with a syringe takes some skill. People who have poor eyesight or unsteady hands can have problems doing injections. If it is difficult for you to do injections, there are aids that can help you.

First, consider using an insulin pen instead of a syringe. (See "Insulin Pens," page 80.) These small devices are convenient and easy to use. If you choose to use a syringe, there are special types of syringes and tools that can make injections easier. If you have poor eyesight, you may want to try a syringe magnifier, which enlarges the markings on the syringe barrel, or a dose gauge, which helps you measure an accurate insulin dose (even mixed doses).

If your hands are not very steady, you might try a needle guide and/or vial stabilizer to help you insert your needle into the insulin vial to draw up your dose.

## Insulin pumps

An insulin pump is a battery-powered, computerized device about the size of a pager. You wear it on your belt or in your pocket. Inside the pump is a syringe of rapid- or short-acting insulin with a gear-driven plunger. A thin tube (21 to 43 inches long) is attached to the pump. At the other end of the tube is a needle or catheter. You insert the needle or catheter under your skin—usually in your abdomen or thigh—and tape it in place. Insulin is delivered through the tube and needle or catheter into your body. You "program" the pump to tell it how much insulin you want and when you want it.

You wear an insulin pump pretty much all the time, either inside or outside your clothes. A pump may be waterproof, or it may be removed for showers and swimming.

# SELF-MONITORING OF BLOOD GLUCOSE

One of the best ways to keep track of how well your diabetes care plan is working is to check your blood glucose. Instead of simply saying to yourself, "I feel fine" or "I feel lousy," you take measurements and keep records. Monitoring helps you find out what happens to your blood glucose level when you eat certain foods, do certain exercises, or lose weight. Monitoring is the only way to know what happens to your blood glucose level when you take diabetes pills or insulin, are sick, or are stressed.

The information you get when you monitor can help you decide what to do to take care of your diabetes. Your results may prompt you to eat a snack, take more insulin, or exercise more. Monitoring may alert you to treat high or low blood glucose. Records of your results can help you and your health care team figure out which diabetes pills or insulin work best for you, at what dosage, and at what times.

## Testing Your Blood Glucose

You monitor your blood glucose with a glucose meter. It's important to follow the instructions that come with the product you buy. You'll need a lancet and a clean test strip.

1. Wash your hands with soap and water.
2. Prick the side of your finger with a lancet.
3. Squeeze out a drop of blood.
4. Apply the drop of blood to the test strip.
5. Read your blood glucose number in the window on the meter.
6. Dispose of the lancet the same way you dispose of used syringe needles. (See "How to Dispose of Syringes," page 82.)
7. Record your results.

## When to monitor blood glucose

Talk to your diabetes care provider about the times you should monitor to get the most helpful information. The most common time is before meals. For instance, monitoring 2 hours after a meal lets you see how well your pre-meal insulin dose matched the food you ate. Monitoring at 2 or 3 a.m. tells you if you have low blood glucose at night.

The more you monitor, the more information you will have about your blood glucose. The more information you have, the better able you will be to make decisions that will help you reach your targets and your goals. Here are some times to talk about with your health care team:

- If you manage your diabetes with healthy eating and exercise only, check before you eat breakfast and 1 or 2 hours after a meal.
- If you are taking diabetes pills, monitor once or twice a day. If you monitor once a day, do it before you eat breakfast. If you monitor twice a day, do it first when you get up in the morning, and vary the time of the second test.
- If you are taking insulin, check 2 to 8 times a day, and vary the times you test.

## Most Common Times to Test

Here are some common monitoring times:

- Before breakfast
- Two hours after breakfast
- Before lunch
- Two hours after lunch
- Before supper
- Two hours after supper
- Before bedtime
- At 2 or 3 a.m.

## When to do extra blood glucose checks

There are times when you will want more information than you get from your routine checks. For example:

- When you are trying to find the best dose of diabetes pills or insulin for you

- When you change your exercise program or meal plan
- When you start a new medicine that can affect your glucose level
- When you think your glucose is low or high
- When you are sick
- When you are pregnant
- When you are traveling
- When you have been exercising for more than an hour
- Before and after you exercise
- Before you drive
- Before activities that take a lot of concentration

## Is your meter accurate?

Sometimes you may wonder whether your meter is accurate, especially if it gives you a reading you were not expecting or if its reading and that of a lab do not match. False readings can occur for many reasons. The problem may be with the meter itself, the testing strips, or your testing technique. Here are some steps to take if you think your meter isn't working properly.

### Check the meter

Dirty meters can give false results. The user's manual that came with the meter will say whether you need to clean it and how to clean it. Review the directions for cleaning your meter, or call the meter's maker if you are unsure about the right way to clean your meter.

Calibrate your meter each time you start a new batch of test strips. The chemical mix that is put on test strips differs a little from batch to batch. Each batch of strips may give slightly different results. Calibrating your meter means resetting it so that you still get correct answers. A few meters calibrate themselves. If you don't recall the calibration procedure and/or can't find the instructions that came with your meter, call the meter's maker. You'll find the maker's phone number on the back of most machines.

Your meter should have come with a *control solution*. The control solution contains a known amount of glucose. Run a test using the control solution anytime the meter does not seem to be working right. It's also a good idea to run a test when you buy the meter, when you open a new batch of test strips, and when you change the batteries. Compare the answer you get with what the meter's manual says you should get. If the answers are not close, something is wrong. The meter may be broken, it may need a new battery, or the problem may be with the test strips or your testing technique.

### Check the glucose strips

Confirm that the glucose strips you have will work with your meter. Keep your test strips in a place that is cool and dry. Strips may give false readings if they have been stored in extreme hot or cold temperatures and/or extreme humidity. Your bathroom, for example, can be too humid for your strips. And the glove compartment of your car can be too hot.

Keep strips in the dark (in their vial or foil wrap) until you are ready to use them. When you remove strips, close the rest up right away to avoid exposing them to direct light for any length of time.

Note the expiration date on each vial or package of glucose strips. Be sure to throw away strips that are past their expiration date. Throw them out if they don't look like fresh new strips.

### Check your technique

Study your manual to make sure you are using your meter correctly. Take your meter to your appointments with your diabetes care provider. Have a member of your health care team check how you monitor.

# LOW BLOOD GLUCOSE

Low blood glucose is known as *hypoglycemia*. You may get low blood glucose if you use insulin or take sulfonylureas or meglitinides. If not treated, low blood glucose can cause you to pass out. If left untreated for an extended period of time, low blood glucose can even cause seizure, coma, and death.

There are many causes of low blood glucose. Perhaps you ate less food or carbohydrate than usual. Maybe you delayed or skipped a meal or snack. You might have exercised harder or longer than usual, or your medication dose may have been too large. Perhaps you are sick, or you drank alcohol on an empty stomach.

Many people experience warning signs of low blood glucose. Your own signs may be different from those someone else feels. Learn your early warning signs of low blood glucose. Tell your warning signs to someone who can help you watch out for them. When any of your warning signs occurs, you need to treat low blood glucose right away.

## Warning Signs—Low Blood Glucose

- Anger
- Anxiety
- Blurred vision
- Clamminess
- Clumsiness
- Confusion
- Fatigue
- Headache
- Hunger
- Impatience
- Irritability
- Light-headedness
- Nausea
- Nervousness
- Numbness
- Pale complexion
- Pounding heart
- Sadness
- Shakiness
- Sleepiness
- Stubbornness
- Sweating
- Tension
- Weakness

## How to treat yourself for low blood glucose

You may have heard that a blood glucose level below 70 mg/dl is low. This is the general standard, but some people have symptoms of hypoglycemia with blood glucose levels above 70, and some people don't feel any symptoms even if they are below 70. Talk to your diabetes care provider about what level to look for when you suspect you have low blood glucose. Then follow these steps:

1. Check your blood glucose if you can. If it is below the level you've set with your care provider, go to steps 2 and 3. If you can't check, go to steps 2 and 4.
2. Eat or drink something with about 15 grams (1/2 ounce) of carbohydrate. Foods with close to 15 grams of carbohydrate are listed above.
3. Wait 15 minutes, and then test again.
4. If your blood glucose is still below the level, repeat steps 2 and 3. If you have repeated steps 2 and 3 and your blood glucose is still low, call your diabetes care provider, or have someone take you to a hospital emergency room. You may need help to treat your low blood glucose.

### Foods That Treat Low Blood Glucose

- Glucose tablets or gel (the dose is printed on the package)
- 1/2 cup (4 ounces) of fruit juice
- 1/3 can (4 ounces) of a regular (not diet) soft drink
- 1 cup (8 ounces) of skim milk
- 2 tablespoons of raisins (40–50)
- 3 graham crackers
- 4 teaspoons of granulated sugar
- 6 saltine crackers
- 6 1/2-inch sugar cubes

## How to have someone else treat your low blood glucose

Sometimes you will not be able to treat low blood glucose your-self. Maybe you did not notice your warning signs, or maybe low blood glucose has made you too confused to treat yourself. Whatever the reason, teach someone else *ahead of time* to do it.

Keep foods to treat low blood glucose near you at all times. Place a small box of juice in your desk drawer at work or at school. Put glucose tablets or gel in your purse or coat pocket and in the glove compartment of your car. Tell others where you keep them.

If you are unconscious, glucagon is your emergency treat-ment for hypoglycemia. *Glucagon* is a hormone that is normally made in the pancreas that raises blood glucose. The ADA recommends that glucagon be prescribed for anyone who is at risk of severe low blood glucose. Glucagon needs to be injected and comes in a kit that you can carry with you. It is a good idea to teach someone you are around frequently to administer glucagon; however, if no one around you is comfortable giving you the injection, make sure they know to call 911 immediately.

### Helping in an Emergency Situation

If you are conscious but cannot swallow:

1. Have someone call 911.
2. Have someone moisten his or her fingertip, dip the fingertip in table sugar, and rub his or her sugar-coated fingertip against the inside of your cheek until the sugar dissolves, being careful to keep the finger away from your teeth. (If you go into a seizure, you may bite the finger.)

OR

3. Have someone open a tube of cake frosting and insert the open end inside your cheek. Have the person squeeze a small amount of frosting into your mouth and massage the outside of your cheek.
4. Keep doing step 2 or 3 until the ambulance arrives.

# HIGH BLOOD GLUCOSE

High blood glucose is known as *hyperglycemia*. High blood glucose is one of the signs of diabetes. Having high blood glucose for a long time can damage your eyes, kidneys, heart, nerves, and blood vessels.

There are many causes of high blood glucose. Maybe you ate more carbohydrate than usual. Perhaps your dose of diabetes pills or insulin is too small, or you forgot to take your medication. You might be sick or feeling stressed. Maybe you weren't able to exercise.

High blood glucose is harder to sense than low blood glucose. If your glucose is very high, you may feel some of the signs listed below. You may not be able to tell that your glucose is too high by signs alone. The only sure way to know is to test your blood glucose. Your glucose reading will help you decide what to do.

Usually, hyperglycemia is defined as blood glucose levels of 250 mg/dl or above. Talk to your diabetes care provider ahead of time to find out what you should do if you develop hyperglycemia. Here are some recommendations:

- If your blood glucose is close to 250 mg/dl, and you have no other symptoms, call your diabetes care provider. You may be advised to exercise a little, drink plenty of fluids, and just wait a little while to see if your levels go down.
- If your blood glucose is between 250 and 350 mg/dl, and you have symptoms of *diabetic ketoacidosis* or *HHS* (see page 92), call your health care team immediately.
- If your blood glucose level is above 350 mg/dl, even if you do not have other symptoms, call a member of your health care team right away.
- If your blood glucose is over 500 mg/dl, call for emergency help or have someone take you to the emergency room at once.

## Warning Signs—High Blood Glucose

- Thirst
- Frequent urination
- Feeling "not right"
- Tiredness
- Lack of energy
- Blurry vision

# Diabetic ketoacidosis (DKA)

People with type 1 diabetes are more likely to get diabetic ketoacidosis (DKA), but it can happen in people with type 2 diabetes, too. DKA occurs when blood glucose levels are consistently in the hyperglycemic range—250 mg/dl and above. If your blood glucose level is above 250 mg/dl, check for ketones in your blood. The body begins to break down fat and protein to get energy for the cells, because there isn't enough insulin to get energy from the glucose in the blood. When fat is broken down, it releases chemicals called *ketones*. DKA occurs when these ketones build up in the blood. It can cause breathing problems, shock, pneumonia, seizures, coma, and even death.

Symptoms of DKA are listed in the box below. If you feel any of these symptoms, check your blood glucose level right

## Warning Signs—Diabetic Ketoacidosis (DKA)

- Lack of appetite
- Stomach pains
- Nausea
- Vomiting
- Blood glucose of 250 mg/dl or above
- Blurry vision
- Fever
- Difficulty breathing
- Flushed sensation
- Weaknesses
- Drowsiness
- Intense thirst
- Dry mouth
- Need to urinate frequently
- Fruity odor on your breath

away. If it is at 250 mg/dl or above, call your diabetes care provider immediately.

## Hyperosmolar Hyperglycemic Syndrome (HHS)

HHS is an abbreviation for hyperosmolar hyperglycemic syndrome. It is a life-threatening condition of high blood glucose and severe dehydration. Anyone with type 2 diabetes can develop HHS, but it is most common in people who don't use insulin. HHS doesn't just happen—it is usually brought on by something else, such as stress, an infection, or a heart attack or stroke.

In HHS, blood glucose levels rise, and your body tries to get rid of the excess glucose by passing it into your urine, making your urine thicker. Fluids are pulled from all over your body to thin out the urine. You make lots of urine, and you have to urinate more often. You also get very thirsty. If you don't drink enough fluids at this point, you can get dehydrated.

If HHS continues, the severe dehydration will lead to seizures, coma, and eventually death. HHS usually takes days or even several weeks to develop, which is why its particularly important for you to drink lots of fluids when you are sick. When you are sick, drink a glassful of fluid (alcohol-free) every hour, and check your blood glucose more often.

### Warning Signs—HHS (Hyperosmolar Hyperglycemic Syndrome)

- Blood glucose level over 350 mg/dl
- Dry, parched mouth
- Extreme thirst (although this may gradually disappear)
- Warm, dry skin that does not sweat
- High fever (105°F, for example)
- Sleepiness or confusion

# MONITORING BY YOUR HEALTH CARE TEAM

Your health care team will monitor your health and how well your treatment plan is working. How often you need to see members of your health care team will depend on your health, your blood glucose goals, and any changes that need to be made to your diabetes care plan. The chart below will give you an idea of when to visit your health care providers and what tests to expect.

Most people with type 2 diabetes have two regular checkups a year. Regular checkups help your health care team detect problems as early as possible. During a physical exam, members of your health care team will check your:

- Height and weight
- Blood pressure and pulse
- Hands and fingers
- Eyes
- Feet
- Mouth, teeth, and gums
- Skin
- Neck
- Nervous system
- Heart

Sometimes, your health care team will order laboratory tests, such as an A1C test to measure your average blood glucose level for the past two to four months, or a blood fat (lipid) profile to measure your total cholesterol, LDL cholesterol, HDL cholesterol, and triglycerides. (For sample A1C measurements, see the table on page 95; for sample lipid profile values, see the "Blood Fats (Lipid) Profile" table in Chapter 5.)

## Sample A1C Measurements

| A1C Measurement (%) | Estimate Average Glucose (eAg) (mg/dl) |
|---|---|
| 6 | 126 |
| 7 | 154 |
| 8 | 183 |
| 9 | 212 |
| 10 | 240 |
| 11 | 269 |
| 12 | 298 |

## Recommended Frequency of Medical Exams and Tests

| | Every 3 Months | Every 6 Months | Every Year | Every 2–3 Years | As Needed |
|---|---|---|---|---|---|
| **Regular Visits*** | | | | | |
| If not meeting goals | I | | | | |
| If meeting goals | | I | | | |
| **Physical Exam** | | | I | | |
| **Dilated Eye Exam** | | | I | | |
| **Lipid Profile** | | | | | |
| If last reading was abnormal | | | I | | |
| If last reading was normal | | | | I | |
| **Glycohemoglobin Test** | | | | | |
| If not meeting targets or if treatment changes | I | | | | |
| If meeting targets | | I | | | |
| **Kidney Tests** | | | I | | |
| **Urine Tests** | | | I | | |
| **Thyroid Tests** | | | | | I |
| **Electrocardiogram** | | | | | I |

*Regular visits include measurement of your height, weight, and blood pressure, a foot exam, an eye exam, and a check on anything that was abnormal at a previous visit.

# CHAPTER 5

# Diabetes Complications

Diabetes can lead to other related health conditions called *diabetes complications*. Complications can affect your blood vessels, heart, brain, legs and feet, eyes, kidneys, and nerves. These complications are caused by untreated higher-than-normal levels of blood glucose over time.

Your diabetes care plan can help you keep your blood glucose level close to normal and can help prevent complications. It is a good idea to be familiar with the types of complications diabetes can cause, so you know what symptoms to look for and understand how diabetes touches so many areas of your health.

## BLOOD VESSELS

High blood glucose, high blood pressure, high blood fats (cholesterol and triglycerides), and cigarette smoking can damage your blood vessels. Often, you will not notice any signs until the damage has been done.

When blood vessels are damaged, they become weak, narrow, or blocked. This is called *atherosclerosis,* or hardening

## Coping With Complications

If you have a complication, learn all you can about it. The more you know about your complication, the more in control you will feel.

- **Talk with family and friends.** Tell them what's going on and what they can do to help.
- **Seek counseling.** If you find it hard to talk with family and friends, you may want to get counseling from a social worker or psychologist.
- **Join a support group.** Other people who have diabetes or complications can give you support. Your diabetes care provider or the local ADA office may be able to help you find a support group (*www.diabetes.org*).
- **See a specialist.** Think about going to a specialist who deals with your complication. Your diabetes care provider should be able to refer you to one.
- **Ask questions about treatments.** What are the treatments? What are the side effects of the treatments? How much do these treatments cost? How often will I need treatments? How many patients with this problem have you treated?
- **Try to get a second opinion.** Check your health insurance. It might cover a second opinion.
- **Look for organizations that focus on your complication.** Organizations like the National Kidney Foundation, the American Foundation for the Blind, the Neuropathy Association, and the National Amputation Foundation have programs and services. For more information, see "Resources," page 159.

of the arteries. Less blood flows through the blood vessels to nourish the parts of your body with oxygen. When your body parts get less oxygen, they don't work as well and can become damaged or die.

Quitting smoking is one way to protect your blood vessels. Medications, meal planning, and exercise can also help lower your blood glucose, blood pressure, and blood fats.

# HEART

Decreased blood flow to your heart can cause pain in your chest during exertion (angina). The pain goes away after resting a minute or so. Angina is a signal that your heart muscle is working hard but not getting enough blood for its effort.

Angina may be relieved by drugs (such as nitrates, including nitroglycerine; beta-blockers; calcium-channel blockers; and vasodilators) that increase the amount of oxygen going to the heart or reduce the amount of oxygen the heart needs when it's working hard. Surgery may be needed when these treatments are not working or when a heart attack is likely to occur.

Despite decreased blood flow to the heart, some people with diabetes may not have chest pain. Some may even have a severe heart attack and not feel pain. This can happen when the nerves to the heart have become damaged; **nerve damage** is another diabetes complication. (See "Nerves," page 107.)

A heart attack occurs when blood flow to part of the heart is stopped. Blood flow can be cut off by a buildup of fat and cholesterol in the blood vessels. This condition is called *atherosclerosis*. During a heart attack, part of the heart muscle dies or is damaged.

If you have suffered a heart attack caused by a blockage in an artery, you may need surgery. There are several different types of surgery that doctors use to repair an artery blockage. In arterial bypass surgery, a healthy vein is taken from another part of the body and sewn onto the blocked artery above and below the blockage. Blood then flows around the

## Warning Signs—Heart Attack

- Prolonged pain, tightness, pressure, or squeezing in the chest
- Pain that spreads to the neck, shoulders, arms, or jaw
- Shortness of breath or hiccups
- Sweating
- Nausea
- Dizziness or fainting

**Note:** If you have nerve damage to your heart or your nerves, you may not feel pain.

blockage. In laser angioplasty, a laser beam melts the blockage. In balloon angioplasty, the narrowed part of the artery is stretched by an inflated balloon. To keep the artery open, the surgeon may insert a stent, which is like a small, rigid pipe. In *atherectomy,* a blocked artery is opened by boring a hole through the blockage.

# BRAIN

As explained above, heart attacks are caused when a buildup of fat and cholesterol in the blood vessels block the flow of blood. When this happens in a blood vessel that leads to the brain, it instead causes an *ischemic stroke.* This is the most common type of stroke.

Sometimes, the blood flow to the brain is blocked only for a brief time. This is called a *transient ischemic attack,* or TIA. TIAs may pass quickly because your body releases enzymes that dissolve the clot and restore blood flow. If you have TIAs often, you are more likely to have a major ischemic stroke.

Another type of stroke is a *hemorrhagic stroke.* It occurs when a blood vessel in your brain leaks or breaks. The most common cause of hemorrhagic strokes is high blood pressure.

If you have had an ischemic stroke, you may be given drugs to prevent new clots from forming or to keep an existing clot from getting bigger. Occasionally, surgery (a carotid endarterectomy) is performed to remove a blockage from the

## Warning Signs—Stroke or TIA

- You are suddenly weak or numb in your face, an arm, or a leg.
- Your sight is suddenly dim, blurred, or lost.
- You can't speak or can't understand someone else who is talking.
- You have a sudden headache.
- You feel dizzy or unsteady, or you suddenly fall.

carotid artery in the neck. For a hemorrhagic stroke, you may be given drugs to reduce blood pressure.

# LEGS AND FEET

You've learned that high blood glucose can damage blood vessels, which carry blood to all parts of the body. Healthy blood vessels keep the blood moving through the body at all times. When blood vessels are damaged, blood can't circulate through the body like it should.

Damage to the blood vessels that circulate blood through the legs and feet can be particularly dangerous. Poor circulation in the legs and feet can make it difficult for wounds in these areas to heal. It also makes it easier for wounds in the legs to become infected.

Antibiotics can help prevent wounds from becoming infected. Also, in the early stages, blood vessel disease can be treated with exercise, drugs, or surgery to open blocked blood vessels. Possible surgeries include arterial bypass surgery, laser angioplasty, balloon angioplasty, or atherectomy.

In serious cases, poor circulation can starve leg and foot tissues of oxygen. Sometimes, this can cause tissues in the legs and feet to die. This is called *gangrene*. If dead tissues in the legs and feet become infected with bacteria, doctors may have

## Symptoms—Blood Vessel Damage to the Legs and Feet

- Cramping or tightness in one or both legs while walking, known as *intermittent claudication*
- Cold feet
- Pain in the legs or feet while at rest
- Loss of hair on the feet
- Shiny skin
- Thickened toenails

to operate to remove the dead tissues. This may mean amputation of all or part of a foot or leg.

# EYES

Like other parts of your body, your eyes depend on blood flow to stay healthy. Over time, high blood glucose can weaken the blood vessels that lead to the eye. This can impact different parts of the eye and cause different types of vision problems. The three eye diseases that people with diabetes develop most often are *retinopathy, cataracts,* and *glaucoma.* Of the three, retinopathy is the most common.

Often, these eye diseases can develop without any symptoms; however, if they are found early, there are treatments that can help protect your sight. That's why it is important for people with diabetes to visit an eye care specialist for an eye exam. Your eye care specialist should do a dilated eye exam to check your eyes for diabetes complications.

## Retinopathy

The retina is the lining at the back of the eye that senses light. Small blood vessels called *capillaries* bring oxygen to the retina. Over time, high blood glucose levels damage these small blood vessels. As a result, the retina gets less oxygen than it needs, and blood vessels enlarge in an attempt to get more. The two major types of retinopathy are *nonproliferative* and *proliferative.*

### Nonproliferative retinopathy

In nonproliferative (or background) retinopathy, the small blood vessels in the retina bulge and form pouches, called *microaneurysms.* This weakens the blood vessels, and they may leak a bit of fluid. This leaking does not usually harm your sight. Often, the disease never gets worse.

If the disease does get worse, the weak blood vessels leak a larger amount of fluid, along with blood and fats. This causes the retina to swell. The swelling will usually not harm your sight, unless it occurs in the center of the retina.

The center of the retina is called the *macula*. The macula helps you see fine details. Swelling in the macula is called *macular edema*. Macular edema can blur, distort, reduce, or darken your sight.

Nonproliferative retinopathy is found in one of every five people who are diagnosed with type 2 diabetes. Most people with type 2 diabetes do not go on to develop proliferative retinopathy.

### Proliferative retinopathy

In proliferative retinopathy, the capillaries are so damaged that they close completely. In response, many new, very small blood vessels grow in the retina. As these new blood vessels grow, they branch out to other parts of your eye.

These changes may not affect your sight, or they may reduce your peripheral vision. You might also find it harder to see in the dark and to adjust from light to dark.

The new blood vessels are fragile. They may break and bleed into the clear gel that fills the center of the eye. This is known as a *vitreous hemorrhage*. The most common signs of vitreous hemorrhage are blurring and floating spots. If not treated, vitreous hemorrhage can cause you to lose your sight.

Broken blood vessels may cause scar tissue to form on the retina. Scar tissue can wrinkle the retina and pull it out of place. A retina that has been pulled away from the back of the eye is a *detached retina*. A detached retina will cause you to see a shadow or large dark area. It can endanger your sight.

Diabetic retinopathy can be treated successfully if it is found early. The best-known treatment for retinopathy is *laser surgery*. A laser is used to make tiny burns in the retina. This

## Symptoms: Retinopathy

- Your sight gets blurry.
- You see floating spots.
- You see a shadow or dark area.
- You can't see things on either side of you.
- You have trouble seeing at night.
- You have trouble reading.
- Straight lines do not look straight.

Usually, you can't see the early signs of damage to your retina, but your eye care specialist can. That's why it is important for people with diabetes to have an eye exam every year.

patches up leaky vessels, destroys the extra blood vessels, and discourages new fragile vessels from growing.

Macular edema can also be treated with laser surgery. In addition, low-vision aids, such as magnifying lenses (for close-up) and telescopic lenses (for distance) may be helpful.

When there is a vitreous hemorrhage or a detached retina, a *vitrectomy* may be needed. A vitrectomy is an operation to remove broken blood vessels and scar tissue, to stop bleeding, to replace some of the vitreous fluid within the eye with a salt solution, and, sometimes, to repair the detached retina.

## Cataracts

A cataract clouds the eye's lens. The lens is usually clear and lies behind the iris (the colored part of your eye) and the pupil (the dark opening). The lens focuses light onto the retina. Clouding of the lens blocks light from entering. Cataracts usually start out small. Some of them never bother your sight. Others block most or all of your sight. How a cataract will affect your sight depends on three things: 1) how large it is, 2) how thick it is, and 3) where it is on the lens. Because of these three things, signs that you have a cataract may vary.

Cataracts are common in older people, whether they have diabetes or not. But cataracts can occur at younger ages in people with diabetes.

Cataracts can be treated with surgery. The clouded lens is removed and replaced with a clear, plastic lens.

## Symptoms—Cataracts

- Your sight is hazy, fuzzy, or blurry.
- You think you need new glasses.
- Your new glasses don't help you see any better.
- You find it harder to read and do other close work.
- You blink a lot to see better.
- You feel you have a film over your eyes.
- You feel you are looking through a cloudy piece of glass, veils, or a waterfall.
- Light from the sun or a lamp seems too bright.
- At night, headlights on other cars cause more glare than before or look double or dazzling.
- Your pupil, which is usually black, looks gray, yellow, or white.
- Colors look dull.

## Glaucoma

Glaucoma is a buildup of fluid in the eye. The fluid buildup causes increased pressure, which can damage your optic nerve. Your optic nerve tells your brain what your eye sees. Fluid can build up when the filter it normally drains out of becomes clogged. There are two kinds of glaucoma: *chronic open-angle glaucoma* and *acute angle-closure glaucoma*.

### Chronic open-angle glaucoma

Chronic open-angle glaucoma is the most common type of glaucoma. It develops when fluid pressure in the eye rises slowly over many years. You usually won't notice it. You might feel the increased pressure in your eye, or your eyes may keep tearing. As glaucoma worsens, you may notice that your sight is slightly blurry or foggy, or that you have a hard time seeing in the dark. If not treated, you may lose your sight.

### Acute angle-closure glaucoma

Acute angle-closure glaucoma is a less common type of glaucoma. It occurs when fluid pressure in the eye builds up quickly. Your eyes will probably hurt and will probably be blurry and tear up frequently. You may see colored halos around bright lights. You may even vomit. If you have any of these signs, go to a hospital emergency room right away. Glaucoma is treated with prescription eye drops or pills that decrease the amount of fluid the eye makes.

## KIDNEYS

Your kidneys clean your blood by letting wastes pass into the urine. Kidney disease, or *nephropathy,* is damage to the small blood vessels in the kidneys that do the cleaning. Overworked, weak blood vessels may start to leak a protein called *albumin.* One job of albumin is to hold water in the blood. If there is not enough albumin in the blood, water leaks out of the blood vessels. The water can end up in the ankles, the abdomen, and the chest, which is called *edema.* Water in these places can be the first physical sign that something is wrong with your kidneys.

But many people don't have any physical signs that they are developing kidney disease, which is why people with type 2 diabetes should have a *microalbumin test* each year. This test, performed by your health care provider, checks your urine for albumin. Even a small amount of albumin in the urine can be a sign of kidney damage. Another test that can be done to determine the amount of kidney damage and the stage of kidney failure is the estimated *glomerular filtration rate* (GFR).

People with type 2 diabetes are more likely to develop kidney disease if they also have high blood pressure. The combination of high blood glucose levels and high blood pressure can overwork and weaken the blood vessels in the kidneys. At the early stages, kidney disease is treated by focusing on these two things: blood glucose levels and blood pressure. Weight loss, exercise, and changes like giving up smoking and cutting back on salt and alcohol may be recommended to help blood pressure. There are also medicines that can help bring blood pressure down.

If the damage to the blood vessels continues, eventually the kidneys can't do their job, and wastes build up in the bloodstream. This is kidney failure or *end-stage renal disease*. When this occurs, dialysis can be used to filter out wastes, or a kidney transplant can provide new, healthy kidneys.

## Symptoms—Kidney Failure

- Foul taste
- Poor appetite
- Upset stomach
- Throwing up
- Easy bruising

- Restless legs
- Loss of sleep at night
- Fatigue during the day
- Lack of concentration
- Water retention

# NERVES

Nerve damage, or *neuropathy*, is very common in people with type 2 diabetes. Neuropathy can affect any of the *peripheral nerves*, that is, all the nerves in your body except for nerves in the brain and spinal cord.

There are three types of peripheral nerves: *motor, sensory,* and *autonomic. Motor nerves* control voluntary muscle movement. *Sensory nerves* allow you to feel and sense. *Autonomic nerves* control involuntary activities, like digestion, and they also allow you to receive signals, such as that of a full bladder. For men, these are nerves involved in getting an erection. There are many types of neuropathy.

## Distal symmetric polyneuropathy

Distal symmetric polyneuropathy is nerve damage to the feet and legs and sometimes the hands. It is the most common form of neuropathy. People with this type of neuropathy may have numbness or loss of feeling; muscle weakness; tingling or prickling sensations; shooting or stabbing pain; pain on contact with bed sheets or clothing; the sensation of bugs crawling over the skin; or the sensation of walking on a strange surface.

The major goal of treatment for distal symmetric polyneuropathy is pain relief. Lowering your blood glucose levels can help. There are also medications for neuropathy to ease the symptoms. Other pain relief options include TENS (transcutaneous electrical nerve stimulation) and capsaicin topical cream.

### Get a Foot Exam

Make sure your health care provider does a full foot exam annually to determine if there is any damage to the foot. A foot exam will consist of:

1. A test to determine if you have adequate sensation in your feet.
2. Looking at the bone structure and how you walk.
3. A check for blood flow by checking your pulses and feeling your skin temperature.
4. Observing the skin for signs of decreased blood flow and feeling.

## Charcot foot or joint

Charcot foot, also called *neuropathic arthropathy,* usually starts with a loss of feeling in the foot, sudden swelling, redness, and warmth. But what you may notice first is that you can't get your shoe on. If you have these symptoms, keep your weight off the foot and call your doctor immediately. Early treatment for Charcot foot is crucial; if you continue to walk on the foot, bones in the arch and ankle will fracture and collapse. This will cause a deformed foot.

Early treatment can stop the breakdown of bone and promote healing. The foot is usually put into a cast for three to four months. This keeps the joint from moving and keeps weight off the foot. Later, as the foot heals, you can wear extra-depth or custom-molded shoes. Surgery may be able to restore a deformed foot.

## Cranial neuropathy

Cranial neuropathy affects the nerves that control sight, eye movement, hearing, and taste. It can cause facial pain and temporary paralysis of eye muscles or parts of the face. It usually goes away without treatment.

## Autonomic neuropathy

Autonomic neuropathy can affect the nerves that control your heart, lungs, blood vessels, stomach, intestines, bladder, and sex organs.

### Heart, lungs, and blood vessels

Nerve damage to your heart, lungs, and blood vessels can affect your heart rate and blood pressure. Your heart may pound hard and fast even when you are at rest. You may get dizzy or feel faint when you stand up quickly. This is because your blood pressure drops. Your blood pressure may go up when you are sleeping and down when you are standing. You may have a painless heart attack.

Prescription medications can control your blood pressure. In addition, you can try to stand up slowly when you get out of bed, avoid standing for long periods, and elevate your head when you sleep.

### Stomach

Nerve damage to your stomach can affect digestion by delaying the stomach's ability to empty. You may feel bloated, even after a small meal, and sick to your stomach. You may vomit food that you ate more than one meal before. Treatment may involve eating six or more small liquid meals; eating more high-fiber, low-fat foods; and taking prescription medications that stimulate the stomach to empty.

### Intestines

Damage to nerves in your intestines can cause diarrhea or constipation, sometimes alternating. These conditions can be relieved by prescription or over-the-counter medications that your health care provider recommends. Drinking more water and eating more high-fiber foods may be all that is needed for constipation.

### Bladder

If the nerves in your bladder are damaged, you will not be able to tell when your bladder is full of urine. You may dribble or wet yourself. The urine that stays in your bladder may lead to a urinary tract infection.

Treatment of this condition usually requires that you urinate every 3 or 4 hours when you are awake, even if you feel as if you don't need to. After you urinate, press down on the lower abdomen to help empty the bladder. Other treatments include use of a catheter, prescription medications, and surgery.

### Sex organs

Nerve damage to the sex organs can cause erectile dysfunction in men and vaginal dryness and loss of sensation in women. Erectile dysfunction can be treated in several ways: with drugs; with use of external erection aids, such as a vacuum that pulls blood into the penis; or with penis implants. Vaginal dryness can be treated with over-the-counter or prescription lubricants or creams.

## Compression mononeuropathy

Compression mononeuropathy occurs when a single nerve is damaged. It is a fairly common type of neuropathy. There seem to be two kinds of damage. In the first, nerves are squashed at places where they must pass through a tight tunnel or over a lump of bone. Nerves of people with diabetes are more prone to compression injury. The second kind of damage arises when blood vessel disease caused by diabetes restricts blood flow to a part of the nerve.

Carpal tunnel syndrome is probably the most common compression mononeuropathy. It occurs when the median nerve of the forearm is compressed at the wrist. Symptoms of this type of neuropathy include numbness, swelling, or prickling in the fingers—with or without pain—when driving a car, knitting, or resting at night. Simply hanging your arm by your side usually stops the pain within a few minutes. If the symptoms are severe, an operation can give complete relief from pain.

# BLOOD PRESSURE

People with diabetes are more likely to have high blood pressure, or *hypertension,* than people without diabetes. High blood pressure usually has no symptoms. The only way to know if you have high blood pressure is to get it checked. Your blood pressure should be checked each time you visit your diabetes care provider.

Blood pressure is reported as two numbers. The first number is the *systolic pressure.* Systolic pressure is the force of your blood when your heart contracts. The second number is the *diastolic pressure.* Diastolic pressure is the force of your blood when your heart relaxes.

A reading of "130 over 80" means a systolic pressure of 130 and a diastolic pressure of 80. It is written as 130/80 mmHg (millimeters [mm] of mercury [Hg]). This is the recommended blood pressure level for people with diabetes.

If you find out that your blood pressure is high, you and your health care team can take steps to control it. Your health care team will first try to find out the cause of your high blood pressure.

Sometimes, there is a specific cause, such as a kidney problem, hormone disorder, pregnancy, or the use of birth control pills. When high blood pressure is linked to a specific cause, it is called *secondary hypertension*. If you have secondary hypertension, the first step is to treat the cause.

Most of the time, there is no obvious cause for high blood pressure, which is called *essential hypertension*. If you have essential hypertension, there are things you can do to bring your blood pressure down.

Some people can lower their blood pressure by losing weight. Some people can lower blood pressure by cutting salt in their diet or avoiding alcohol. Because of the risks of having high blood pressure along with diabetes, blood pressure drugs are usually used along with these lifestyle changes.

Blood pressure drugs used most often in people with diabetes are ACE (angiotensin-converting enzyme) inhibitors, alpha$_1$-receptor blockers, calcium antagonists, and thiazide diuretics in small doses.

These blood pressure drugs do not raise blood glucose levels, but they all have side effects. Ask your diabetes care provider or pharmacist about them.

## BLOOD FATS

Blood fats include cholesterol and triglycerides. People with diabetes often have high blood fat levels. High blood fat levels put you at higher risk for heart attack and stroke. People with

## Blood Fats (Lipid) Profile (in mg/dl)

| | Targets for people with diabetes |
|---|---|
| LDL Cholesterol | Under 70 |
| HDL Cholesterol | Women: above 50 mg/dl<br>Men: above 40 mg/dl |
| Triglycerides | Under 150 mg/dl |

diabetes should have their blood fat levels checked at least once a year to help prevent heart-related complications.

## Cholesterol

There are two main types of cholesterol, and blood tests can tell you how much of each type you have in your blood. This is helpful because one type is dangerous, while the other is beneficial.

The dangerous type of cholesterol is called *LDL cholesterol,* which stands for low density lipoprotein. You may have heard LDL cholesterol called "bad cholesterol," because it is the type of cholesterol that narrows or blocks your blood vessels the most. Blocked vessels can lead to a heart attack or a stroke.

Keeping your LDL cholesterol low protects your heart. People with diabetes should aim to keep their LDL levels at 70 or less. Reaching your LDL cholesterol target first will help you the most. It may be easier to remember this by telling yourself that the "L" in "LDL" stands for "low."

The helpful type of cholesterol is called *HDL cholesterol,* which stands for *high density lipoprotein.* HDL is sometimes called "good cholesterol," because it helps remove deposits from the insides of your blood vessels and keeps your blood vessels from getting blocked. Keeping your HDL cholesterol high helps protects your heart. It may be easier to remember this by telling yourself that the "H" in "HDL" stands for "high."

Target HDL levels are different for men and women. That's because the female hormone estrogen tends to make HDL levels higher. As women get older and produce less estrogen, their HDL levels tends to go down. Older women are at higher risk for heart attack and stroke. Women should try to keep their HDL cholesterol level above 50, while men should aim to keep HDL above 40.

Cholesterol levels are written as mg/dl, which stands for "milligrams per deciliter". Cholesterol levels can be expressed in several different ways. *Total cholesterol* is one number, in the hundreds. It tells you the total amount of all types of cholesterol in your blood.

## Triglycerides

*Triglycerides* are another type of blood fat. High levels of triglycerides can lead to heart attack and stroke. Triglyceries are also written in terms of milligrams per deciliter, or mg/dl. People with diabetes should try to keep their triglyceride levels below 150 mg/dl.

## Medications for blood fats

Most people with diabetes take medications to lower their blood fat levels. The most common type of cholesterol-lowering drugs are called *statins*. There are many different types of statins. If you need medication to bring down your cholesterol levels, you and your health care provider can select one that is best for you. Most people can take statin drugs without side effects; the most common side effects are muscle and stomach pain. Also, statin drugs can affect the liver, so people taking them need to have liver tests once a year.

Sometimes statins help lower triglycerides, as well. If you need extra help lowering your triglycerides, there are medicines for that, too.

## Lower Your Blood Fat Levels

In addition to medications, there are other things you can do to help lower your blood fat levels:

- Lower your A1C to target.
- Lose weight if you need to.
- Replace saturated fats with unsaturated or monounsaturated fat.
- Eat fewer foods high in saturated and trans fat.
- Eat more foods high in fiber.
- Exercise regularly.
- Quit smoking.

# CHAPTER 6

# Lifestyle

## EMPLOYMENT

People with diabetes may be discriminated against (treated unfairly) in the workplace. Discrimination can occur in any aspect of employment, including application procedures, hiring, training, pay, benefits, promotions, tenure, leaves of absence, layoffs, and firings.

Whether you are looking for a job, waiting for a promotion, or deciding whether to tell your employer that you have been diagnosed with diabetes, the first step toward getting fair treatment is to know your rights.

You don't have to tell a potential employer that you have diabetes; however, if you decide to talk about your diabetes during an interview, emphasize the positive. Refer to any awards you've won in previous jobs or other examples of your hard work and good skills. If you haven't used much sick leave, point that out, too.

A potential employer cannot ask you about your health or make you get a physical exam before offering you a job. Some jobs require all employees to get a physical exam after they are hired.

If you have to get an employment physical exam, don't change your treatment plan right before the exam. Changes in routine can affect your blood glucose and blood pressure levels. Be aware that the company's doctor is probably not a specialist in diabetes care. You may want to point out the steps you take to manage your diabetes. For some jobs, you may be required to show that you have good blood glucose levels, and to set up a plan for managing your diabetes to prevent low glucose levels on the job. The employer is allowed to take back a job offer because of the results of a medical exam—but only if the reason is related to the job.

If you are not required to tell your employer about your diabetes as part of a medical exam or licensing process, then whether or not you tell is completely up to you; however, there are some advantages to telling your employer and/or your co-workers. Being open about your diabetes can show others that people with diabetes are safe and responsible workers. If you take insulin, it may help you if your co-workers know how to recognize, and perhaps treat, low blood glucose. Also, if you need to make changes in your work schedule because of your diabetes, your employer may be more understanding of your needs.

Another important reason to tell people is that this is the only way your employment rights will be protected by the Americans with Disabilities Act. The Americans with Disabilities Act is a civil rights law that protects the employment rights of people with diabetes who are considered disabled. You are considered disabled if one of these statements is true:

- Diabetes greatly limits one or more of your major life activities. Some major life activities include, but are not limited to, seeing, hearing, speaking, walking, breathing, doing manual tasks, learning, caring for yourself, and working.

## Discrimination on the Job

Job discrimination can be hard to prove. If you think an employer has discriminated against you because of diabetes, follow these steps:

- Try solving the problem by talking directly with the employer.
- Get the help of a union or employee group.
- Talk to a lawyer. With a telephone call or letter, a lawyer may be able to resolve the problem quickly, making a lawsuit unnecessary.
- File charges with the Equal Employment Opportunity Commission (EEOC), your state anti-discrimination agency, or for federal workers, your agency's Equal Employment Opportunity Office. You must file a charge before going to court, and the time limits to do so are very short. You can reach the EEOC at 1-800-669-4000.
- If you are asked to leave your job, look for other work. If your case goes to court, the court may want to see that you can and want to work.

If you win your case, the employer usually must place you in the position you would have had, give you back pay (the sum of wages that you've lost) and other damages, and pay your costs and lawyers fees.

- You have a record of a disability because at one time, diabetes greatly limited one or more of your major life activities.
- Your employer regards you as disabled because you have diabetes. It does not matter how your diabetes has actually affected you.

Under this law, your employer cannot discriminate against you if you are qualified for the job and if you can do the job with or without "reasonable accommodation." Accommodation means that your employer makes changes in your work, work area, or schedule or provides equipment or training to help you do the job. The employer is required to make accommodations unless it would cause an "undue hardship" because it is very difficult or expensive to do.

Employers do not have to give you more sick leave than other workers; however, under the Family and Medical Leave

Act, you may be entitled to 12 weeks of unpaid leave per year to deal with your own or a close family member's diabetes care. This leave can be taken in small blocks of time.

In addition, employers do not have to give you preference over other equally qualified people who apply for the job. They can choose whoever they feel can best perform a job.

If you are rejected for a position, ask for a written explanation. Keep copies of the job announcement and your job application. Make notes of your conversations and meetings with potential employers, including dates, times, places, names of those present, and the subjects discussed.

The Americans with Disabilities Act applies to private companies, state and local governments, employment agencies, and labor unions. The Act does not apply to employers with fewer than 15 workers, Native American tribes, tax-exempt private clubs, or the federal government. People who work for the federal government or for organizations that get federal funds are protected by the Federal Rehabilitation Act of 1973. In addition, all states have their own employment rights laws. Some of these laws provide even more protection than the federal laws.

The American Diabetes Association can provide more information about employment discrimination. Visit *www. diabetes.org* and search on "employment discrimination," or call the ADA at 1-800-DIABETES (342-2383).

## TRAVEL

Your diabetes should not keep you from traveling. You can go anywhere you want to go. It just takes planning to manage your diabetes while you are away from home. How you prepare will depend on where you are going, how you are getting there, and how long you will be there.

## Planning ahead

There are a few things you should do before any type of trip:

- Get a medical exam. You and your health care provider can discuss any questions you may have about managing your trip, and your health care provider can make sure there aren't any issues developing that could be a problem.
- Ask your diabetes care provider to put together a letter saying that you have diabetes. The letter should also list any medications that you take, such as diabetes pills or insulin, or devices that you use, such as a blood glucose meter or syringes. It should also point out any allergies or adverse reactions to food and medications you may have.
- If you use medication, get a prescription from your health care provider for your insulin or diabetes pills. Even if

### What to Pack

Pack twice as much medication and blood-testing supplies as you think you'll need, because it's always better to have too much than not enough. Pack half in a bag that you'll keep with you at all times. Other stuff to pack in this bag includes:

- The letter from your diabetes care provider stating that you have diabetes
- Prescriptions for diabetes pills, insulin, and other medications
- Diabetes pills
- Insulin
- Syringes, insulin pens, or pump supplies
- Other medications
- Glucose meter
- Test strips
- Lancets
- Glucose tablets or gel
- Snacks, such as cheese and crackers, juice, fruit, peanut butter, bagels, and baby carrots

you don't need a prescription in your state, you may need one in other states or foreign countries. Be prepared, so you'll always be able to get insulin, syringes, or diabetes pills if you need them.

- Get a medical I.D. (identification) bracelet or necklace that indicates that you have diabetes, and wear it at all times while traveling.

## Car travel

If you are traveling by car, make sure you stick to your care plan schedule of monitoring, medication, and meals. Don't forget about time changes if you cross time zones.

If you use insulin, be sure to pack it in bags that protect it from extreme heat or cold. In the summer, keep insulin in an insulated container with ice in a bag or "blue ice" (but don't allow the insulin to freeze), a cool damp cloth, or some other cooling agent. Your automobile glove compartment and trunk can get too hot. Backpacks and cycle bags also can get quite hot in direct sunlight. Consider buying a special travel pack to protect your insulin while you are away from home.

## Air travel

Traveling by airplane requires some extra planning. In the world of increased airport security, you'll need to take some extra steps to make sure you get to your plane on time and protect your supplies.

Always pack your diabetes medications and supplies in a carry-on bag, just in case your luggage gets lost. This means that your medications and supplies will be subject to additional screening by security. The ADA and the Transportation Security Administration (TSA) have worked together to provide guidelines for traveling with diabetes supplies. When you reach airport security, notify the screener that you have diabetes and are carrying your supplies with you.

## Tips to Make Airline Travel Easier

- Insulin and insulin-loaded dispensing products must be clearly identified with a prescription label containing a name that matches the passenger's name on his or her ticket.
- If you live in a state where a prescription is not required for regular insulin, it must be clearly labeled.
- You may carry up to 3 ounces of liquids and gels to treat hypoglycemia. If containers are more than 3 ounces, passengers need to declare these items to security checkpoint personnel.
- You may carry an unlimited number of unused syringes when accompanied by insulin or other injectable medication.
- You can carry blood glucose meters, blood glucose meter test strips, continuous blood glucose monitors, lancets, alcohol swabs, meter-testing solutions, and monitor supplies.
- You may use an insulin pump and can carry insulin pump supplies (cleaning agents, batteries, plastic tubing, infusion kit, catheter, and needle).
- You may carry urine ketone test strips.
- You may carry an unlimited number of used syringes as long as they are in a Sharps disposal container or other similar hard-surface container.

If you need to inject insulin during your flight, remember to consider the time zone changes as you fly. Here is a rule of thumb: Eastward travel results in a shorter day, so if you inject insulin, less insulin may be needed. On the other hand, traveling west gives you a longer day and may require more insulin. If you have concerns about insulin adjustment while crossing time zones, take your round-trip airline flight schedule to your diabetes care provider along with information on the time zone changes. Work out the appropriate adjustments for travel days. These may depend on your meal schedule and plans for sleep or activity on arrival at your destination. Self-monitoring of blood glucose while traveling will help you make informed decisions.

Pressure differences in the airplane can make it more difficult to fill a syringe using your usual method. Avoid injecting air into the insulin bottle, which can make it harder to move the plunger and measure insulin accurately. Consider using an insulin pen for in-flight doses. Also, food is rarely available on flights these days, and delays are to be expected. Plan ahead and pack snacks and/or meals in your carry-on bag that fit in with your meal plan. For more information, visit *www.tsa.gov*.

## Traveling overseas

If you have to get special vaccinations to prepare you for your destination, have them at least one month before you leave. This will give you time to even out any effects the shot may have had on your glucose levels.

It's a good idea to learn how to say, "I have diabetes" and "Sugar or orange juice, please" in the languages of the areas you will be visiting. Write the phrases down to carry with you. You can point to them if you have trouble pronouncing them.

Before you go, contact the International Diabetes Federation to find a group in the areas you will be visiting (see resources). You may also want to request a list of English-speaking foreign health care providers from the International Association for Medical Assistance to Travelers. (See "Resources," page 159.) If an emergency occurs while you're traveling and you don't have a list, contact the American Consulate, American Express, or local hospitals for a list of health care providers.

# EATING OUT

Today, more and more people eat at restaurants. Restaurant owners have become more health-conscious. Most restaurant menus now feature "lite" or "healthy" entrees. All eating places offer sugar substitutes and diet beverages, while many have reduced-calorie salad dressings, low-fat or skim milk, and salt substitutes. It's also easier to find salads, fish and seafood, vegetables, baked or broiled food, and whole-grain breads.

More restaurants are offering menus that list calories and nutrients or provide the information on request. If you ask,

## Table Tips for Eating Out

- If you can, pick a restaurant that offers a variety of choices.
- If you don't know the ingredients in a dish or the serving size, ask.
- Try to eat the same size servings that you eat at home. If the servings are too large, use a doggie bag before you start eating, or share portions with your dining partner.
- Eat slowly. Take the time to savor each bite.
- Ask that fish or meat be broiled with little added fat.
- Ask that sour cream or butter for the baked potato be put on the side or left off.
- Ask that sauces, gravy, and dressings be served on the side.
- Use the menu creatively. For instance, order the fruit cup appetizer or the breakfast melon for your dinner dessert.
- Ask for substitutions, such as low-fat cottage cheese, baked potato, or even a double portion of a vegetable instead of French fries.
- Ask about low-calorie items, like salad dressings, even if they're not listed on the menu.
- Substitute low-calorie or calorie-free beverages for alcoholic beverages.

chefs can adjust food preparation for you. Some cooks will remove the skin from a chicken, omit extra butter on the dish, broil instead of fry, and serve sauces on the side. There are restaurants that will allow you to order small portions at reduced prices. If you like the choices on a restaurant's menu, let the manager know. If you'd like to see more low-calorie, low-cholesterol choices on the menu, say so. Restaurants, like any business, only know what you want if you tell them.

## Eating on time

If you take diabetes pills or insulin, ordering the right foods isn't your only concern. You need to think about when you eat as well. Eating around the same times each day helps keep your blood glucose levels more even.

- If you're eating with others, ask whether they would mind eating at your usual time.

- Try to avoid the busiest hours at the restaurant, so you are less likely to have to wait.
- Ask whether special requests will take extra time to be prepared and served.
- If your meal is going to be later than usual, eat a piece of fruit or bread at your usual mealtime.
- If dinner will be very late, eat your bedtime snack before dinner.

## Making healthy choices when eating out

| | Choose | Avoid |
|---|---|---|
| Appetizers | Tomato juice or other juice<br>Raw vegetables<br>Fresh fruit, unsweetened<br>Fresh steamed seafood<br>Clear broth, bouillon, consomme | Cream soups, thick soups<br>Marinated vegetables<br>Canned fruit cocktail<br>Breaded or fried seafood |
| Eggs | Poached or boiled | Fried, creamed, or scrambled |
| Salads | Tossed vegetable<br>Cottage cheese | Coleslaw<br>Canned fruit or gelatin salads |
| Breads | Whole-grain rolls, crackers, breads | Sweet rolls, coffee cake, croissants |
| Potatoes, Pasta, Rice | Baked, boiled, or steamed potatoes<br>Steamed rice or pasta | Fried, French fried, creamed,<br>  scalloped, or au gratin potatoes |
| Fats | Low-calorie salad dressing<br>Low-fat sour cream or yogurt | Regular salad dressing<br>Regular sour cream<br>Gravy, cream sauces |
| Vegetables | Raw, stewed, steamed, or boiled | Creamed, scalloped, or au gratin |
| Meat, Poultry, and Fish | Roasted, baked, or broiled<br>Lean meats with skin or fat<br>  removed | Fried, battered, or breaded<br>Cured meats, organ meats<br>Stews and casseroles<br>Gravy, cream sauces |
| Desserts | Fresh fruit<br>Non-fat or low-fat frozen yogurt | Sweetened fruit<br>Pudding, custard, pastries |
| Beverages | Coffee, tea<br>Skim milk<br>Diet soda<br>Water | Chocolate milk, cocoa<br>Milk shakes<br>Regular soft drinks |

# Fast food

Today's fast-food restaurants are offering healthier choices—such as salads, baked potatoes, chili, and grilled chicken—that make it easier to fit fast food into your meal plan. There are still plenty of high-fat, high-calorie fast-food choices out there. Be careful what you order. It is possible to eat an entire day's worth of fat, salt, and calories in just one fast-food meal.

## Tips for Fast Food Eating

- For breakfast, try a whole-grain bagel, toast, or English muffin with peanut butter. Order pancakes without butter, or plain scrambled eggs. Avoid bacon and sausage.
- Load up on lettuce and vegetables at a salad bar. Go easy on the dressing, bacon bits, cheeses, croutons, and pasta salads. Try cottage cheese or salsa instead of dressing. Add garbanzo or kidney beans for added carbohydrate and protein.
- Order regular or junior-size sandwiches rather than the larger "jumbo," "giant," or "deluxe" sandwiches to get fewer calories and less fat, cholesterol, and sodium.
- Skip the cheese or croissant, and eat your sandwich on a bun or bread instead to save calories and fat.
- Choose chicken or fish if it is roasted, unbreaded, grilled, baked, or broiled without fat.
- Stay away from double burgers or super hot dogs with cheese, chili, or sauces. Cheese can carry an extra 100 calories, as well as extra fat and sodium.
- Order items plain without toppings or rich sauces. Add lettuce, tomato, onion, and mustard instead.
- Choose cheese pizza with vegetables. **A word of caution:** Pizza can make blood glucose levels go really high in some people. The high fat content of pizza may delay the blood glucose rise until several hours later. Check your blood glucose at different times after eating pizza to learn how it affects you.
- Order tacos, tostados, bean burritos, soft tacos, and other non-fried items when eating Mexican foods. Choose chicken over beef. Avoid beans refried in lard. Pile on extra lettuce, tomatoes, and salsa. Go easy on cheese, sour cream, and guacamole.
- If you have room for dessert, go for sugar-free non-fat frozen yogurt. Ices, sorbets, and sherbets have less fat and fewer calories than ice cream, but they are high in sugar. Some places now offer fresh fruit!

You may be counting calories, grams of carbohydrate, or grams of fat. Keep these general rules in mind: Eat a variety of foods in moderate amounts, limit your fat intake, and watch the amount of sodium in your food choices.

Many fast-food restaurants can give you the nutritional information on their food if you ask. By knowing the nutritional value of fast-food items, you can choose foods that will fit into your meal plan. If you have fast food for one meal, try to include low-fat foods and more fruits and vegetables for your other meals that day. Eating out can be one of life's great pleasures. By balancing the meals you eat out with the meals you eat at home, you can enjoy yourself and take care of your diabetes at the same time.

# ALCOHOL, DRUGS, AND TOBACCO
## Alcohol

One or two drinks a day will have little effect on your blood glucose level as long as you are free of complications and drink the alcohol close to or with a meal. Drinking two drinks on an empty stomach, however, can cause low blood glucose if you are taking diabetes pills or insulin, or if you were just exercising or about to exercise.

Usually, if your blood glucose drops too low, your liver puts more glucose into the blood. (The liver has its own supply

## Tips to Cut Alcohol Calories

- Use 80 proof in place of 100 proof alcohol. The lower the proof number, the less alcohol in the liquor. Each gram of alcohol has seven calories.
- Put less liquor in your drink.
- Use no-calorie mixers, such as diet sodas, club soda, or water.
- Choose light beer over regular beer.
- Choose dry wine over sweet or fruity wines and wine coolers.
- Try a wine spritzer made with a small amount of wine and a lot of club soda.

# Nutritional Content in Alcoholic Beverages

| Beverage | Serving (ounces) | Alcohol (g) | Carbohydrate (g) | Calories |
|---|---|---|---|---|
| **Beer** | | | | |
| Regular | 12 | 13 | 13 | 150 |
| Light | 12 | 11 | 5 | 100 |
| **Distilled spirits, 80 proof** (gin, rum, vodka, whiskey, scotch) | 1 1/2 | 14 | Trace | 100 |
| **Dry brandy, cognac** | 1 | 11 | Trace | 75 |
| **Table wine** | | | | |
| Dry white | 4 | 11 | Trace | 80 |
| Red or rose | 4 | 12 | 2 | 85 |
| Sweet wine | 4 | 12 | 5 | 105 |
| Light wine | 4 | 6 | 1 | 50 |
| Wine cooler | 12 | 13 | 30 | 215 |
| Nonalcoholic wine | 4 | Trace | 6–7 | 25–35 |
| **Sparkling wines** | | | | |
| Champagne | 4 | 12 | 4 | 100 |
| Sweet kosher wine | 4 | 12 | 12 | 132 |
| **Appetizer/dessert wines** | | | | |
| Sherry | 2 | 9 | 2 | 74 |
| Sweet sherry, port, muscatel | 2 | 9 | 7 | 90 |
| Cordials, liqueurs | 1 1/2 | 13 | 18 | 160 |
| **Vermouth** | | | | |
| Dry | 3 | 13 | 4 | 105 |
| Sweet | 3 | 13 | 14 | 140 |
| **Cocktails** | | | | |
| Bloody Mary | 5 | 14 | 5 | 116 |
| Daiquiri | 2 | 14 | 2 | 111 |
| Manhattan | 2 | 17 | 2 | 178 |
| Martini | 2 1/2 | 22 | Trace | 156 |
| Old Fashioned | 4 | 26 | Trace | 180 |
| Tom Collins | 7 1/2 | 16 | 3 | 120 |
| **Mixes** | | | | |
| Mineral water | Any | 0 | 0 | 0 |
| Sugar-free tonic | Any | 0 | 0 | 0 |

*(continued)*

## Nutritional Content in Alcoholic Beverages *(Continued)*

| Beverage | Serving (ounces) | Alcohol (g) | Carbohydrate (g) | Calories |
|----------|------------------|-------------|------------------|----------|
| Club soda | Any | 0 | 0 | 0 |
| Diet soda | Any | 0 | 0 | 0 |
| Tomato juice | 4 | 0 | 5 | 25 |
| Bloody Mary | 4 | 0 | 5 | 25 |
| Orange juice | 4 | 0 | 15 | 60 |
| Grapefruit juice | 4 | 0 | 15 | 60 |
| Pineapple juice | 4 | 0 | 15 | 60 |

of glucose, called *glycogen.*) But when alcohol is in the body, the liver wants to get rid of it first. While the liver is taking care of the alcohol, your blood glucose may drop to dangerous levels.

To avoid low blood glucose, always have something to eat when you have a drink. Check your blood glucose before, during, and after drinking. Alcohol can lower blood glucose for as long as eight to 12 hours after your last drink.

Alcohol on your breath may mislead people into thinking you are drunk, and you may not get the treatment you need for low blood glucose. If you drink and then drive when you have low blood glucose, you may be pulled over for drunk driving. When you drink, let someone else drive.

If you treat your diabetes with diet and exercise, low blood glucose when drinking is less likely to happen. Work with a dietitian to include your favorite drink in your meal plan. Be aware that regular beer, sweet wines, and wine coolers will raise your blood glucose more than light beer, dry wines, and liquors (such as vodka, scotch, and whiskey) because they contain more carbohydrate.

Alcoholic beverages supply lots of calories (anywhere from 60 to 300 calories each) but few nutrients. You'll need to add the calories from alcoholic drinks to your daily calorie count.

## Cooking with alcohol

When alcohol is heated in cooking, either on top of the stove or in the oven, some of it evaporates. How much of it evaporates depends on how long you cook it. If you cook it for 30 minutes or less, about one-third of the alcohol calories will remain.

# Drugs

Certain medications raise your blood glucose, others lower it. If you take prescription or over-the-counter medications or choose to use illegal drugs, understand that they may affect your blood glucose levels.

## Caffeine

Caffeine is found in coffee, tea, chocolate, and many soft drinks. Caffeine may raise your blood glucose level slightly. Other side effects include not being able to sleep, shaking, and increased blood pressure and heart rate. You could confuse your reaction to caffeine with the symptoms of low blood glucose.

# Tobacco

Smoking or chewing tobacco is especially dangerous for people with diabetes. Smoking increases your risk of having heart disease and blood vessel disease. Chewing tobacco increases your risk for oral cancer.

There are nicotine-replacement products that can help you quit smoking. Nicotine patches, gum, and lozenges put a small amount of nicotine into your blood, which lets you taper off from the physical addiction slowly. Be careful, because nicotine patches can raise blood glucose levels in people with diabetes. If you are interested in trying nicotine replacement, talk about it with your diabetes care provider before starting.

## Tips to Help You Quit Smoking

Here are a few suggestions that might help you quit smoking, courtesy of the National Cancer Institute:

- List all the reasons why quitting is a good idea.
- Each day, decide how many cigarettes you will smoke.
- Decide when you will quit, and then do it.
- Don't put yourself into situations where you "usually" smoke until your resolve is strong.
- Talk to your health care provider about aids to help you stop smoking.

Some people find it easier to quit with a group of people. Your company, health plan, or a local hospital may sponsor a quitting support group, or the American Lung Association, and the American Cancer Society may run free or low-cost classes in your town. (The American Heart Association and the American Lung Association also have self-help materials. (See "Resources," page 159.) Check your phone book for the local affiliates in your area, and look in the Yellow Pages under Smokers Information & Treatment Centers.

# CHAPTER 7

# Finding the Best Care

As you've learned, diabetes is a disease that you can learn to manage day by day by yourself. That doesn't mean that you will be alone in the process. Along the way, you will build a team of health care providers and other professionals who will help you. Think of yourself as the captain of this team. It is important for you to choose your team members carefully. You want providers who can give you with the best-quality care and advice and who you feel comfortable working with for the long term.

## YOUR HEALTH CARE TEAM

A health care team is a group of health care professionals who help you manage your diabetes. You are the most important member of the health care team. Only you can do the exercising, follow the meal plan, take the medication, and monitor the results. You'll be the first to notice any problems. You're also likely to be the first to take action. All team members will rely on you to tell them how your diabetes care plan is working and when you need their help.

Your health care team may include, at one time or another, your diabetes care provider, a nurse, a dietitian, a mental health professional, an exercise physiologist, an eye doctor, a foot doctor, a dentist, a pharmacist, and other specialists as needed.

## Your diabetes care provider

You will likely communicate with your diabetes care provider more than any other member of your care team, so it's especially important to choose well. Look for a health care provider with experience in diabetes. (See "Certified Diabetes Educator," page 141.) You may choose an internist, a family practitioner, a general practitioner, a nurse practitioner, or a physician's assistant who cares for people with diabetes. You may also be able to choose an endocrinologist or a diabetologist. An *endocrinologist* is a medical doctor who has special training and certification in treating diseases such as diabetes. A *diabetologist* is a medical doctor who has a special interest in diabetes.

You'll also want to think about the type of person you are and the type of people you like to work with. Care providers are people, too, and they each have their own styles and personalities. Think about how you work with others in your life and how those patterns may influence your diabetes care team.

If you are looking for a diabetes care provider, you might check with friends or relatives who have diabetes and are satisfied with their medical care, get referrals from health care professionals you know and trust, or try a referral service sponsored by your local hospital or a professional medical society. (See "Resources," page 159.)

If possible, schedule an appointment just to talk with the provider. Most providers charge for this time, so be sure to ask about the "interview" fee. During the interview, take time to look over the office. Do you feel comfortable with the staff? How long are you kept waiting past your appointment time? Are educational materials on display?

## Important Questions to Ask Your Doctor

If you are able to choose from among many care providers, you may consider asking each of them questions like these during the "interview" appointment:

- How many of your patients have diabetes?
- Do you treat more people with type 1 or with type 2 diabetes? How many patients with type 2 diabetes do you see a month?
- Do you know about the ADA Standards of Medical Care for People with Diabetes?
- Will the care you provide and recommend follow those standards?
- Do you work with, or refer to, a certified diabetes educator (CDE) or registered dietitian (RD)?
- How often will regular visits be scheduled? How often will you check my feet and my A1C?
- About how long is an average appointment?
- Who covers for you on your days off?
- What do I do in an emergency?
- Are you associated with other health care professionals so that I can benefit from a team approach?

Communication doesn't always come easily. This can be especially true when you're feeling nervous, worried, or under pressure. Here are some tips for smooth communication between you and your diabetes care provider:

- Before your visit, decide what you want to accomplish, and tell your diabetes care provider at the start of the visit.
- Write down and ask specific questions, if you can. Your diabetes care provider will answer your questions best if he or she clearly understands what you are asking.
- Bring up your emotional concerns and any problems you're experiencing. Don't wait to be asked.
- If your diabetes care provider uses words that are too technical, and you don't understand what is being said, ask for an explanation.

- Ask your diabetes care provider to repeat anything you didn't hear. Take the time to write down information or instructions.
- Remind your diabetes care provider of previous decisions, lab results, annual appointments, or symptoms. It's not fair to expect the provider to remember everything about you from visit to visit.
- If your diabetes care provider offers recommendations that you know you can't or won't follow, say so. There are lots of ways to treat diabetes.
- Consider bringing a support person (spouse or relative) to sit in on the visit. Sometimes, a second pair of ears will hear things a bit differently.

Some diabetes care providers may already have a team you can work with for all of your health care needs. If not, ask for referrals to a dietitian, a nurse, or other medical specialists you want on your team.

## Nurse

You probably won't get to choose a nurse the way you choose your diabetes care provider or your dietitian. Instead, your nurse will be on staff at your diabetes care provider's office. Nurses are an important part of your health care team.

Look for the initials "RN" after a nurse's name. RN stands for *registered nurse*. Some nurses also have a bachelor's degree (BSN) or a master's degree (MSN). Nurses teach and advise you on the day-to-day management of your diabetes.

Nurses can help you understand:

- What diabetes is and how it is treated
- How nutrition, exercise, and stress affect your blood glucose levels

- How to become more physically active
- How medicines can help you manage your diabetes
- How to monitor your blood glucose and how to use the results to reach your targets
- How to prevent, detect, and treat diabetes complications
- How to reduce your risks for diabetes complications
- How to set goals and solve problems that arise
- How to cope with the emotional side of diabetes
- How to plan for and have a healthy pregnancy, if you want to get pregnant

## Dietitian

A dietitian is an expert in food and nutrition. Food is a key part of your diabetes care. A dietitian can work with you to create a personal meal plan based on your food preferences, weight, goals, lifestyle, diabetes treatment, other drugs you may be taking, and your other health goals.

When your weight, lifestyle, or other goals change, your meal plan will need to change, as well. Your dietitian can help you adjust your meal plan to fit your changing life and goals.

Look for the initials "RD" after a dietitian's name. RD stands for *registered dietitian*. A registered dietitian has met standards set by the Commission on Dietetic Registration. An RD may also have a master's degree.

You might see the initials LD after a dietitian's name. LD stands for *licensed dietitian*. Many states require dietitians to have a license.

Medicare and most insurers will cover sessions with a dietitian. Many insurers call this "medical nutrition therapy services" or "MNTS". Medicare covers three hours of one-on-one work with a dietitian in the first year after diagnosis, and two hours each year after that. Check with your insurer to see what they cover.

## What a Dietitian Can Do for You

Dietitians can teach you many useful skills, such as how to:

- Choose a meal planning system
- Use a meal plan
- Find out how the foods you eat affect your blood glucose levels
- Make a sick-day meal plan
- Read food labels
- Choose wisely when grocery shopping
- Choose wisely from restaurant menus
- Turn a high-fat or high-sugar recipe into a low-fat or low-sugar one
- Find cookbooks and food guides
- Find out how the foods you eat affect your blood fat levels
- Treat yourself for low blood glucose

Your diabetes care provider or local hospital may be able to recommend a dietitian. The American Dietetic Association can also refer you to a dietitian. Call their Consumer Nutrition Hot Line at 1-800-366-1655.

## Exercise physiologist

An exercise physiologist is trained in the science of exercise and body conditioning. An exercise physiologist helps you plan a safe, effective exercise program. Look for someone with a master's or doctoral degree in exercise physiology, or find a licensed health care provider who has graduate training in exercise physiology. Certification from the American College of Sports Medicine is a good sign.

An exercise physiologist can show you the safest exercises for you, whether you have arthritis, are overweight, have complications of diabetes, or have been sitting for years and now want to become more active. Always check with your diabetes care provider about any exercise program, to make sure it is safe for you.

## Mental health professional

Mental health professionals include social workers, psychologists, and psychiatrists. All are trained to help you with the emotional side of diabetes, anxiety, and depression. Look for a licensed clinical social worker (LCSW) with a master's degree in social work (MSW) and training in individual, group, and family therapy. Social workers can help you and your family cope with the stress or anxieties related to diabetes. They can help you locate community or government resources to help with medical or financial needs.

A clinical psychologist has a master's or doctoral degree in psychology and training in individual, group, and family psychotherapy.

A psychiatrist is a medical doctor who can provide counseling for the emotional problems and stresses of diabetes and can prescribe drugs to treat these problems.

## Dentist

At first, it may seem odd to think of your dentist as a member of your diabetes care team; however, dentists have the important role of helping you maintain a healthy mouth and strong teeth. High blood glucose increases your risk for gum disease and other mouth infections. It's recommended that you have a dental checkup every six months and to tell your dentist that you have diabetes.

## Eye doctor

Your eye doctor is either an ophthalmologist or an optometrist. Ophthalmologists are doctors who detect and treat eye diseases. They may prescribe eye medicines and perform eye surgery. Optometrists are trained to examine the eye for vision problems and other minor problems.

Your eye doctor will examine your eyes for any changes, determine what those changes mean, and discuss with you how best to treat your eyes. The ADA recommends that you have yearly dilated eye and visual exams.

## Foot doctor

A podiatrist, or foot doctor, is trained to treat foot and lower-leg problems. Podiatrists have a doctor of podiatric medicine (DPM) degree from a college of podiatry. They have also done a residency (hospital training) in podiatry. People with diabetes are at risk for foot problems because minor foot problems can become serious quickly.

The ADA recommends that you have your feet examined at every regular visit by your diabetes care provider. If you or your diabetes care provider find any problems with your feet or lower legs, you may want to see a podiatrist. To find a podiatrist, check with your diabetes care provider, area hospitals, or your local ADA affiliate or chapter. (See "Resources," page 159.)

## Pharmacist

A pharmacist is trained in the chemistry of drugs and how drugs affect the body. A pharmacist has at least a bachelor of science in pharmacy degree (BScPharm) or a doctor of pharmacy degree (PharmD). Your pharmacist can help you in several ways. Most pharmacists offer free counseling. They can tell you:

- How often to take your prescription drugs
- Whether to take your drugs with meals or on an empty stomach
- What side effects to watch for
- What foods to avoid
- What other drugs might react with your new drug

- When to take a missed dose
- How to store your drugs
- What nonprescription drugs work best with your other drugs
- What special precautions are needed

## Certified diabetes educator

The letters "CDE" after a person's name stand for *certified diabetes educator*. When you see these letters, you know the person is specially trained to teach people with diabetes. These letters may come after the names of any of the people on your health care team.

A diabetes educator becomes certified by passing a test offered by the National Certification Board for Diabetes Educators. The test covers medications, monitoring, biological changes and complications, psychosocial issues, and education principles related to diabetes. Once certified, CDEs must stay up to date on diabetes care and treatment, and their license must be renewed every five years. To find a diabetes educator in your area, call the American Association of Diabetes Educators at 1-800-832-6874 or visit them online at *www. diabeteseducator.org*.

# DIABETES EDUCATION CLASSES

A great way to get a solid foundation in diabetes care is to attend a diabetes education program. To learn about local programs, contact the ADA (see "Resources," page 159) or ask your local hospitals, the county or state department of health, or your diabetes care provider. Contact each program and ask for information so you can compare what they have to offer.

Most insurance plans cover diabetes education classes. Medicare covers 10 hours of diabetes education the first year after diagnosis plus an additional two hours each year after that. Medicare and most insurers require that the education program be recognized by the American Diabetes Association. Call the ADA at 1-800-DIABETES or check *www.diabetes.org* to find out which diabetes education classes in your area have achieved recognition.

Many programs will also advertise that they meet the National Standards for Diabetes Self-Management Education Programs. Classes that meet these standards have skilled and experienced health professionals as instructors and are designed to suit your needs. Certified programs must include training in the following subject areas:

- Diabetes disease process
- Nutrition
- Physical activity
- Medications
- Monitoring/using results
- Acute complications
- Chronic complications
- Goal setting and problem solving
- Psychosocial adjustment
- Preconception care, pregnancy, and gestational diabetes

## HOSPITAL STAYS

At some point in your life, you may have to go to the hospital. The reason for going to the hospital might have nothing to do with your diabetes, but it is still important that the hospital staff knows that you have diabetes. As you've learned, diabetes can affect many areas of your health. If you are hospitalized, you may not be able to follow your meal plan, you won't be able to exercise, and you may not get as much rest as you usually do. Medicines and other treatments you are given in the hospital can cause your blood glucose to go up. All that, plus the stress of being in the hospital, can make it hard to keep your blood glucose levels within range.

Having blood glucose levels within range are especially important when you're in the hospital. Research has shown that people with diabetes get better faster, have fewer complications, and spend fewer days in the hospital when their blood glucose levels stay stable and within target range.

Talk to your diabetes care provider now about how to handle a trip to the hospital. Your provider may be able to recommend a local hospital that has experience treating people with diabetes. You can also do some research on your own. Find out if any local hospitals have the Joint Commission's Advanced Inpatient Diabetes Care certification (*www.qualitycheck.org*). The Joint Commission, an independent nonprofit organization that evaluates and accredits health care institutions in the United States, has teamed up with the ADA to provide this certification program to hospitals. To receive the certification, the hospital must show that its staff follows the latest standards of care for people with diabetes while they are in the hospital.

The ADA also issues Standards of Medical Care for Diabetes each year, which include guidelines for caring for people with diabetes in the hospital. These standards have changed significantly in recent years. Before you need to go to the hospital, find out which local hospitals have adopted these new standards.

You'll also want to consider where your diabetes care provider has hospital privileges, and which hospitals are covered by your insurance. Find the answers to these questions now, so that if you suddenly need to go to the hospital, you'll know the best place to go.

Once you're in the hospital, you'll want to notify your diabetes care provider immediately. You may also want to request a consultation with an endocrinologist—a medical

## When You're in the Hospital

Here are some tips while in the hospital. On admission,

- Tell them you have diabetes.
- Give them a list of all medications you are taking, when you take them, and in what dosages.
- Alert them to medications you are allergic to or that cause severe side effects in you.
- Tell them about other medical conditions you have, such as high blood pressure, kidney damage, or eye problems.
- Tell them about any frequent low blood glucose reactions.
- Tell them about your meal plan and any special needs, such as low sodium.
- Alert them to any food allergies you have.

doctor who specializes in disorders like diabetes. An endocrinologist can help make sure that your blood glucose levels stay close to normal while you're in the hospital.

The ADA's new standards of care recommend keeping blood glucose levels quite low during a hospital stay, lowering the risk of complications like infections. It is also important to keep blood glucose levels stable, which can be difficult in the hospital. If you normally take diabetes pills, you may be asked to stop taking them and use short-term insulin while you are in the hospital. Diabetes pills can interact with other medications you are given in the hospital and can make it difficult to manage quick changes in your blood glucose level. Even if you normally take no medication, you may be asked to use short-term insulin while in the hospital. Research has shown that this is the best way to care for people with diabetes in the hospital. This doesn't mean that you will have to keep using insulin once you are out of the hospital; the hospital staff and your diabetes care team will help you switch back to your normal care plan when you are ready to go home.

Many hospitals put patients with diabetes on a bedside glucose monitor to keep track of blood glucose levels. When you are in the hospital, this can be more convenient and easier than trying to remember to monitor your blood glucose yourself. Plus, all the changes and stress of a hospitalization make it necessary to monitor more often. Your care team will help you transition back to self-monitoring when you are ready to go home.

## When you're facing surgery

Anesthesia and other drugs you may be given before, during, and after surgery can affect your blood glucose levels. Research shows that people with diabetes have better results after surgery when their blood glucose levels are low and stable before, during, and after the operation. It's especially important that your surgeon and anesthesiologist know that you have diabetes, and that they work with an endocrinologist to make a plan before your surgery.

Emergency surgery aside, your first question may be whether the surgery is necessary. There are times when you may want to get a second opinion before proceeding with surgery. Consider getting a second opinion when:

- A provider recommends surgery, long-term medication, or other treatments
- You have doubts about the recommendation or just want reassurance from another provider
- Your health insurance company insists on a second opinion before paying full coverage for certain treatments or surgery

When you are searching for a health care provider to give a second opinion, ask a health care provider you trust. Try calling the appropriate department of a major medical

## Questions to Ask Before Surgery

- Why do you suggest surgery for me?
- What is the success rate of the surgery?
- What does the surgery involve?
- What are the risks of the surgery? What are the side effects? How likely are they to happen?
- What will happen if I do not have the surgery?
- Who will do the surgery?
- How long will I be in the hospital?
- Will there be restrictions on my activities after surgery? For how long?
- When can I go back to work?
- Will I need follow-up care, such as repeated blood tests, physical therapy, or skilled nursing care?

center or teaching hospital. Ask for the name of a specialist in the field.

# HOME HEALTH CARE

If you are bedridden with a long illness or housebound for a short time, you may want some of the services provided by home health care agencies. These include nursing care; physical, respiratory, occupational, or speech therapy; chemotherapy; dialysis; nutrition and diet therapy; personal care, such as bathing and dressing; and homemaker care.

Home health care agencies may provide blood testing or bring a nurse into your home to administer drugs and other treatments. Home health care agencies include the Visiting Nurses Association, the Veterans Administration, nonprofit public agencies run by city or county health departments, nonprofit private agencies, and for-profit agencies operated by individuals or by corporations. If you are looking for home health care, ask for help or recommendations from your friends, family, diabetes care provider, local ADA affiliate, or local hospital.

## Questions to Ask Home Health Care Agencies

Once you get the names of agencies, call or visit them, and consider asking the following questions:

- How soon can services begin?
- Are services available seven days a week, 24 hours a day if needed?
- Must I sign up for a minimum number of hours?
- Will a detailed care plan be prepared before services begin?
- Can I interview potential nurses or aides before they are assigned? Is there a fee for this?
- Can I request a change in nurse or aide?
- What are the fees for various services?
- Will the agency submit bills directly to my insurance company/Medicare/Medicaid?
- Will I get a copy of these bills?
- How often are bills sent?

# NURSING FACILITIES

If you require more care, there are several other options. **Assisted living facilities** offer help with activities of daily living, like dressing, bathing, and getting around. Staff are on hand 24 hours a day, but they have little or no medical training. Residents have private rooms and a lot of independence.

If you require more care, a **skilled nursing facility** or **nursing home** is one option. Skilled nursing facilities can provide medical care (medication, rehabilitation), personal care (help with eating, bathing, dressing), and residential services (room, food, social activities). RNs and MDs are available 24 hours a day.

If you are looking for an assisted living or skilled nursing facility, consult the same sources you would for home health care (see page 146). Once you have found several nursing facilities, call and ask them to send an information packet. Schedule a visit to the facilities that offer the kind of care you seek. You may want to take along a family member or a friend. The more eyes the better.

# HEALTH INSURANCE

Caring for your diabetes can be costly, so finding the best possible health insurance coverage is important. Look for a health insurance plan that meets your health care needs as well as your budget. Health insurance plans vary on what they will cover. Before you sign up for a health insurance plan, find the answers to these questions.

If you already have a health insurance plan, call your benefits manager and find out what diabetes-related items and services your plan does and does not cover. Ask about each item you use. If your plan covers "durable medical equipment," then it may pay for a blood glucose meter, a fingerstick device, an insulin pen or syringes, and an insulin pump, if prescribed by your diabetes care provider as "medically necessary." If your plan covers prescription medications and/or medical supplies, then it may pay for insulin, lancets, glucose meter strips, ketone test strips, and insulin pump supplies, if you have a prescription for them.

Your diabetes care provider may have to provide a thorough explanation in writing of why each of these items is necessary for you. Keep a copy of this explanation because it serves as your "prescription" for these items.

If you believe that your insurance carrier is not covering things that it is supposed to, contact your state insurance department. Each state has its own laws and regulations governing insurance. Many states have legislation that determines insurance coverage for people with diabetes.

## Group coverage

If you work, your employer may offer you a group health insurance plan. Group plans are usually open to all employees.

## Questions to Ask About Health Insurance

- Are visits to my diabetes care provider covered?
- Is there a limit on how many times I can see my diabetes care provider in a year?
- How much will I have to pay per visit?
- How much will the plan pay for a hospital stay?
- Is there a limit on what I pay each year?
- Is there a limit on what the plan pays each year?
- Will I be covered right away, or will I have to wait because I have diabetes (a pre-existing condition)?
- Does the plan cover blood glucose meters, strips, insulin, syringes, pens or pumps, and other diabetes supplies?
- Does the plan cover diabetes education?
- Does the plan cover dietitians, mental health professionals, and specialists?
- What prescriptions are covered? Is there a prescription plan to reduce costs? How often can prescriptions be refilled? What is the co-payment for each prescription?
- Is home health care covered? Are there any limitations?
- Is long-term care covered?

Your employer may pay most or all of the cost (premium) for you. For an additional fee, these plans may also cover your spouse and children.

If your employer does not offer health insurance, you may still be able to obtain group health insurance through membership in a professional, trade, or religious association. Benefits vary widely, so be sure to find out what they are.

If you are self-employed, contact your state department of health or insurance commission to find out whether your state offers a small-business purchasing pool or a high-risk insurance pool. The cost of insurance pools varies widely among the states, although most try to keep it affordable by placing limits on the premium. There are also several small-business associations, such as the American Business Association, that offer health insurance to members and their employees.

## Individual coverage

If you are not eligible for any form of group health insurance, try to find an affordable individual health insurance policy. Although it can be difficult, it is a necessity for people with diabetes. (See "The Health Insurance Portability and Accountability Act of 1996," page 152, for more on individual health insurance policies.)

## Fee-for-service plans

In a fee-for-service plan, you and/or your employer pay a yearly fee to an insurance company. The insurance company then pays for all or part of the cost of your medical care. Usually, the insurance company will start paying after you have paid a small amount of the cost, called a *deductible.*

Many health care providers expect you to pay the total fee at the time of service. You must then apply to your insurance company to receive your reimbursable expenses. Sometimes the provider or hospital will accept assignment of benefits, meaning that they will wait for your insurance company to pay its share and then bill you for the remainder.

The biggest advantage of a fee-for-service plan is that you pick the health care providers you want to go to.

### Health maintenance organizations (HMOs)

An HMO is an organization that hires or contracts with health care professionals to provide a wide range of medical services to individuals and families. Most of the cost of your medical care is covered by a fee paid by you and/or your employer.

Depending on the type of HMO, you may or may not have to satisfy a deductible and/or pay a co-payment at each visit. You may or may not be covered if you go to a provider who is outside the HMO. Before you sign up, be sure to find out how the HMO works.

### Preferred provider organizations (PPOs)

A PPO is a list of health care providers. The list is prepared and provided by an insurance company. The providers on the list are "preferred" because they have agreed with an insurer to discount their fees.

The preferred providers are paid by the insurer and by a small co-payment from you when you go to them. You may have to pay a small deductible. You may choose to go to a provider who does not belong to the PPO, but you will pay more out of your own pocket.

### Exclusive provider organizations (EPOs)

An EPO is like a PPO with an important difference: If you choose to go to a provider who does not belong to the EPO, you pay the total bill.

## COBRA

COBRA stands for *Consolidated Omnibus Budget Reconciliation Act*. This federal law lets some people keep their health insurance coverage for a limited time when they would otherwise lose it. You may need health insurance coverage when you are between jobs, when you go from full-time to part-time status, or when you retire. Your dependents may need health insurance coverage if you die or if you and your spouse separate or divorce.

COBRA allows you and your covered dependents to stay covered under your employer's group health insurance plan. Private companies and state and local government offices participate in COBRA. Employers with fewer than 20 employees, the federal government, and churches are not covered.

If you want to stay covered, you must notify your employer in writing within 60 days of the event that will cause you to lose coverage. Coverage begins the day you would have lost health insurance. Coverage may last for up to 18 months after you leave your job. If you are disabled, coverage may last up to 29 months. Your dependents may keep coverage for up to 36 months.

You pay the share of the premium you paid before, usually along with your employer's share, and a small service fee as well. This is almost always less expensive than purchasing a new short-term policy. When your coverage is over, your employer may allow you to convert to an individual policy. Individual coverage is costly, but this option keeps you insured. For more information on COBRA, call the COBRA Hot Line at 202-219-8776.

## The Health Insurance Portability and Accountability Act of 1996 (HIPAA)

The Health Insurance Portability and Accountability Act of 1996, also know as HIPAA, makes it easier for people with diabetes to get and keep their health insurance.

According to the Act, insurers and employers may not make insurance rules that discriminate against workers because of their health. All workers eligible for a particular health insurance plan must be offered enrollment at the same price.

Insurers who sell individual policies must offer an individual policy without pre-existing condition exclusions to anyone who has had continuous coverage in a group plan for the previous 18 months, is not currently eligible for coverage under any group plan, and has used up COBRA coverage.

If you have had diabetes for more than 6 months and have had continuous coverage by an insurance plan, and then leave your job, you cannot be denied coverage by your new employer because of a pre-existing condition. If, however, you have been recently diagnosed (up to 6 months ago), and you change jobs, your new employer may refuse or limit your health insurance coverage for 12 months. This is a one-time waiting period, and it can be reduced by the number of months you had continuous coverage at your previous job. For example, say you were diagnosed with diabetes while employed and covered by your employer's health insurance plan. Five months after the diagnosis, you change jobs. Your new employer may limit or deny your health insurance coverage for the remainder of the 12-month waiting period, or 7 months.

## Medicare

Medicare is a federal health insurance program for people age 65 and older and for people who cannot work because of certain disabilities. It is run by the Centers for Medicare & Medicaid Services (CMS), an agency of the United States Department of Health and Human Services. Social Security Administration offices throughout the United States take applications for Medicare.

There are four parts to Medicare: Parts A, B, C, and D. Part A and Part B are what some people refer to as "original Medicare." Parts C and D have been added in recent years to provide more options for Medicare-eligible people. For more information on Medicare, call 1-800-MEDICARE (1-800-633-4227). For a free handbook, *Medicare & You,* visit *www.medicare.gov.*

### "Original Medicare"—Part A and Part B

Parts A and B are called "original Medicare" because they were the only options offered when Medicare was first introduced in 1965.

Part A helps to pay bills for medical care provided in hospitals, skilled nursing facilities, hospices, and homes. Medicare will not pay for custodial care provided in a nursing home or private home when that is the only kind of care needed. Custodial care includes help in walking, getting in

## Supplies and Services Covered By Medicare

*Medicare-covered supplies:*
- Blood glucose meters
- Lancets
- Test strips
- Other supplies for the meter
- Insulin pumps
- Therapeutic footwear and shoe inserts

*Medicare-covered services:*
- Foot care (every 6 months; no referral required)
- Glaucoma testing (no referral required)
- Dilated eye exams
- A1C tests
- Flu and pneumococcal shots
- Diabetes education
- Medical nutrition therapy services

and out of bed, bathing, dressing, eating, taking medicines, and other activities of daily living. Most people do not have to pay for Part A coverage.

Part B helps to pay for health provider's services, ambulance services, diagnostic tests, outpatient hospital services, outpatient physical therapy and speech pathology services, and medical equipment and supplies. Most people pay a monthly fee for Part B coverage, based on their income.

Many regular diabetes supplies and services are covered by Medicare. To get coverage for supplies and services, your health care provider must certify in writing that you need all of these items to manage your diabetes. Certain conditions must be met to get coverage for certain supplies like therapeutic footwear and insulin pumps. Make copies of your provider's written statement. Give a copy of it to your pharmacist each time you purchase these supplies so that it can be submitted along with your Medicare claim.

## Supplies and Services *Not* Covered by Original Medicare

- Diabetes pills
- Insulin
- Syringes
- Insulin pens
- Other prescription drugs

- Alcohol swabs
- Eye exams for glasses
- Gauze
- Orthopedic shoes
- Weight-loss programs

Some or all of these supplies and services may be covered by a Medicare Advantage plan and/or a Part D prescription drug plan. (See below.) For more information about Medicare's coverage for diabetes, visit *www.medicare.gov* and download "Medicare Coverage of Diabetes Supplies & Services," or call the Medicare Hotline. (See "Resources," page 159.)

### Part C—Medicare Advantage

Part C, also called *Medicare Advantage,* is an alternative to original Medicare that is available in some parts of the country. It allows eligible people to enroll in coordinated care plans like HMOs, PPOs, and POS plans offered by private insurers. Medicare Advantage plans cover both inpatient and outpatient care, but their specific coverage rules will vary. If you are considering enrolling in a Medicare Advantage plan, be sure to check the coverage it offers for diabetes care.

### Part D

Part D is Medicare's prescription drug plan. Like Part C, it is offered through private insurers, so coverage can vary from plan to plan. It is available to any Medicare-eligible person. Part D covers a portion of the cost of outpatient prescription drugs. For people with diabetes, Part D covers diabetes pills, insulin, syringes, needles, gauze, and alcohol swabs. People who are enrolled in Medicare Part D pay drug costs up to a certain amount, called a deductible. After the deductible has been reached, Part D pays all or part of the costs.

You do not have to enroll in Part D; you should compare Part D coverage with the coverage that original Medicare or a Medicare Advantage plan would offer for your diabetes medications and supplies. Part D plans vary. Each plan has a *formulary*, or list of drugs it will cover. For example, a plan may cover Amaryl, but not Glucotrol. When evaluating Part D plans, be sure to check the plan's formulary to see whether it covers the medications you use.

## Medigap

Medigap plans cover some of the care and services that original Medicare doesn't. Before Part C (Medicare Advantage) and Part D (prescription drug plans) were available, Medigap provided a way to add coverage options to original Medicare.

People who choose original Medicare may still want a Medigap plan. Medigap plans are sold by private insurance companies. The federal government has defined 10 standard Medigap plans. Some plans may not be offered in your state. You can buy a Medigap plan to pay for Medicare deductibles, skilled nursing care, foreign travel emergencies, preventive care, or other costs.

You cannot be denied Medigap coverage if you apply within 6 months of first applying for Medicare Part B. Prices for the same plan vary with insurance companies. Check prices with several insurance companies before you buy a Medigap plan.

For more information about Medigap, visit *www.medi care.gov* and download a copy of the *Guide to Health Insurance for People with Medicare.* You can also request a copy from any insurance company, or call the Social Security Administration at 1-800-772-1213 and ask that it be sent to you.

## Medicaid

If your income is very low, you might be eligible for Medicaid. Medicaid is a federal and state assistance program. Each state has different rules about who can get Medicaid and what it will cover. Call your state's Medicaid office to find out whether you qualify and what health costs are covered.

## Social Security Disability Insurance

If you lose your job because you are disabled, you may be able to get Social Security Disability Insurance. This insurance covers people younger than age 65 who have worked for pay recently and who are now disabled. Social Security has a list of disabilities that qualify for insurance benefits. If you have a disability on that list and earn less than $500 a month, you are considered disabled. The disabilities that are listed include diabetes with certain kinds of neuropathy, acidosis, amputation, or retinopathy. For more information, call the Social Security Administration at 1-800-772-1213.

# Resources

## FOR THE VISUALLY CHALLENGED

**American Council of the Blind**
*www.acb.org*
1155 15th Street NW, Suite 1004
Washington, D.C. 20005
202–467–5081
800–424–8666
202–467–5085 (fax)
E-mail: info@acb.org

Works to improve the well-being of all blind and visually impaired people by: serving as a representative national organization of blind people; elevating the social, economic, and cultural levels of blind people; improving educational and rehabilitation facilities and opportunities; cooperating with the public and private institutions and organizations concerned with blind services; encouraging and assisting all blind persons to develop their abilities; and conducting a public education program to promote greater understanding of blindness and the capabilities of blind people. Publishes *The Braille Forum,* a free monthly national magazine produced in Braille and large print.

## American Foundation for the Blind

*www.afb.org*
11 Penn Plaza, Suite 300
New York, NY 10001
212–502–7600
800–232–5463
E-mail: afbinfo@afb.net

AFB's priorities include broadening access to technology; elevating the quality of information and tools for the professionals who serve people with vision loss; and promoting independent and healthy living for people with vision loss by providing them and their families with relevant and timely resources.

## American Printing House for the Blind

*www.aph.org*
1839 Frankfort Avenue
P.O. Box 6085
Louisville, KY 40206
502–895–2405
502–899–2274 (fax)
800–223–1839
E-mail: info@apg.org

Manufactures textbooks and magazines in Braille, large print, recorded, and computer disc formats. APH also manufactures hundreds of educational, recreational, and daily living products. APH's fully accessible website features information about APH products and services, online ordering of products, and free information on a wide variety of blindness-related topics. One popular feature of the site is the *Louis* Database, a free tool to help locate accessible books available from organizations across the U.S. APH products can be ordered through *Louis*.

**National Association for Visually Handicapped**
*www.navh.org*
NAVH New York City
22 West 21st Street 6th Floor
New York, NY 10010
212–255–2804
212–727–2931 (fax)

NAVH San Francisco
507 Polk Street, Suite 420
San Francisco, CA 94102
415–775–NAVH (6284)
415–346–9593 (fax)
E-mail staffca@navh.org if you live in these Western States:
AK, AZ, CA, CO, HI, ID, MT, NV, NM, OR, UT, WA, WY
E-mail navh@navh.org for the rest of the U.S. or overseas.

Works to help the "hard of seeing" cope with the psychological effects of visual impairment and to provide low-vision services, visual aids, and training to anyone in need of these services. A list of low-vision facilities is available by state. Visual aid counseling and visual aids, peer-support groups, and more intensive counseling are offered at both offices. Some counseling is done by mail or phone. Maintains a large-print loan library.

**National Federation of the Blind**
*www.nfb.org*
1800 Johnson Street
Baltimore, MD 21230
410–659–9314
410–685–5653 (fax)

Membership organization providing information, networking, and resources through affiliates in all states, the District of Columbia, and Puerto Rico. Some aids and appliances available through national headquarters. The Diabetics Action Network, a division of the NFB, publishes a free quarterly newsletter, *Voice of the Diabetic,* in print or on cassette.

**National Library Service (NLS) for the Blind and Physically Handicapped**
*www.loc.gov/nls*
Mailing address:
Library of Congress
Washington, D.C. 20542

Street Address:
1291 Taylor Street, NW
Washington, D.C. 20011
202–707–5100
202–707–0744 (TDD)
202–707–0712 (fax)
888–NLS–READ
(888–657–7323) to connect to a local library
E-mail: nls@loc.gov

Through a national network of cooperating libraries, NLS administers a free library program of Braille and audio materials circulated to eligible borrowers in the United States by postage-free mail.

**Recording for the Blind & Dyslexic**
*www.rfbd.org*
20 Roszel Road
Princeton, NJ 08540
866–RFBD–585 (866–732–3585)

Library for people with print disabilities. Provides educational materials in recorded and computerized form; almost 80,000 titles on cassette. Registration fee required.

**The Seeing Eye, Inc.**
*www.seeingeye.org*
P.O. Box 375
Morristown, NJ 07963
973–539–4425
973–539–0922 (fax)
E-mail: info@seeingeye.org

Offers guide dog training and instruction on working with a guide dog.

# FOR AMPUTEES

**American Amputee Foundation**
*www.americanamputee.org*
P.O. Box 250218
Little Rock, AR 72225
501–666–2523
501–666–8367 (fax)
E-mail: info@americanamputee.org

Provides information, self-help materials, and referral services. An individual AAF membership also entitles the member to a one year's subscription to *Active Living* magazine.

**National Amputation Foundation**
*www.nationalamputation.org*
40 Church Street
Malverne, NY 11565
516–887–3600
516–887–3667 (fax)
E-mail: info@nationalamputation.org

Sponsor of *Amp-to-Amp* program in which a new amputee is visited by an amputee who has resumed normal life. A list of support groups throughout the country is available. Website provides tips for new amputees.

# TO FIND LONG-TERM OR HOME CARE

**National Association for Home Care & Hospice (NAHC)**
*www.nahc.org*
228 7th Street SE
Washington, DC 20003
202–547–7424
202–547–3540 (fax)

Offers free information for consumers about how to choose a home care agency. Has a searchable online directory of home care and hospice agencies.

# TO FIND QUALITY HEALTH CARE

**American Association for Marriage and Family Therapy**
*www.aamft.org*
112 South Alfred Street
Alexandria, VA 22314
703–838–9808
703–838–9805 (fax)

Offers a searchable online directory of marriage and family therapists across the country.

**American Association of Diabetes Educators**
*www.aadenet.org*
100 West Monroe Street, Suite 400
Chicago, IL 60603
800–338–3633
312–424–2427 (fax)
E-mail: aade@aadenet.org

Offers referrals to local diabetes educators and a searchable online directory of diabetes educators.

**American Association of Sex Educators, Counselors, and Therapists (AASECT)**
*www.aasect.org*
P.O. Box 1960
Ashland, VA 23005
804–752–0026
804–752–0056 (fax)
E-mail: aasect@aasect.org

For a list of certified sex therapists and counselors in any state, send request along with a self-addressed, stamped, business-sized envelope. Searchable online directory of certified sex therapists and counselors.

**American Board of Medical Specialties**
*www.abms.org*
1007 Church Street, Suite 404
Evanston, IL 60201–5913
847–491–9091
866–ASK–ABMS (275–2267)

Record of physicians certified by 24 medical specialty boards. Only certification status of physician is available to callers. Directories of certified physicians organized by city of medical practice and alphabetically by physician names are available in many libraries. Searchable online directory of certified physicians.

**American Board of Podiatric Surgery**
*www.abps.org*
445 Fillmore Street
San Francisco, CA 94117–3404
415–553–7800
415–553–7801 (fax)
E-mail: info@abps.org

Referrals to local board-certified podiatrists.

**The American Dietetic Association**
*www.eatright.org*
120 South Riverside Plaza, Suite 2000
Chicago, Illinois 60606–6995
800–877–1600

"Find a Nutrition Practitioner" feature on website provides referrals to local ADA members.

**American Medical Association**
*www.ama-assn.org*
515 North State Street
Chicago, IL 60610
800–621–8335

Online "Doctor Finder" feature provides basic professional information about virtually every licensed physician in the United States. Also provides links to state medical societies, which may be able to refer you to local physicians.

**American Optometric Association**
*www.aoanet.org*
243 N. Lindbergh Boulevard
St. Louis, MO 63141
800–365–2219

Referral to your state optometric association for referral to a local optometrist.

**American Psychiatric Association**
*www.psych.org*
1000 Wilson Blvd, Suite 1825
Arlington, VA 22209–3901
703–907–7300
E-mail: apa@psych.org

Referral to your state psychiatric association for referral to a local psychiatrist.

**American Psychological Association**
*www.apa.org*
750 First Street NE
Washington, D.C. 20002
202–336–5500
800–374–2721
TDD/TTY: 202–336–6123

Referral to your state psychological association for referral to a local psychologist.

**National Association of Social Workers**
*www.socialworkers.org*
750 First Street NE, Suite 700
Washington, D.C. 20002
202–408–8600
800–638–8799

Referral to your state chapter of NASW for referral to a local social worker.

**Pedorthic Footwear Association**
*www.pedorthics.org*
2025 M St., NW, Suite 800
Washington, D.C. 20036
202–367–1145
800–673–8447
202–367–2145 (fax)
E-mail: info@pedorthics.org

Referral to a local certified pedorthist (a person trained in fitting prescription footwear). Searchable online directory of pedorthists.

# FOR MISCELLANEOUS HEALTH INFORMATION

**American Academy of Ophthalmology**
*www.eyenet.org*
P.O. Box 7424
San Francisco, CA 94120
415–561–8500
415–561–8533 (fax)

For brochures on eye care and eye diseases, send a self-addressed, stamped envelope. Searchable online directory of opthalmologists.

**American Heart Association**
*www.americanheart.org*
7272 Greenville Avenue
Dallas, TX 75231
800–242–8721

**MedicAlert Foundation**
*www.medicalert.org*
2323 Colorado Avenue
Turlock, CA 95382
888–633–4298
209–668–3333 from outside the U.S.
209–669–2450 (fax)
E-mail: customer_service@medicalert.org

**National Kidney Foundation**
*www.kidney.org*
30 E. 33rd Street
New York, NY 10016
800–622–9010

For donor cards and information about kidney disease and transplants.

**United Network for Organ Sharing**
*www.unos.org*
P.O. Box 2484
Richmond, Virginia 23218
804–782–4800
804–782–4817 (fax)

For information about organ transplants and a list of organ transplant centers in the U.S.

# FOR TRAVELERS

**Centers for Disease Control and Prevention**
*www.cdc.gov/travel*

Provides travel health information for a variety of destinations and subject areas. Also provides link to *Health Information for International Travel,* also known as the *Yellow Book.* Can order online at *www.cdc.gov/travel* or by phone by calling Elsevier Science at 800–545–2522.

**Travelers' Health Automated Information Line**
877–FYI–TRIP

A division of the Centers for Disease Control and Prevention.

**International Association for
Medical Assistance to Travelers**
*www.iamat.org*
1623 Military Road #279
Niagara Falls, NY 14304
716–754–4883

For a list of doctors in foreign countries who speak English and who received postgraduate training in North America or Great Britain.

**International Diabetes Federation**
*www.idf.org*
1 rue Defaeqz
B–1000 Brussels, Belgium

For a list of International Diabetes Federation groups that can offer assistance when you're traveling.

# FOR EXERCISE INFORMATION

**American College of Sports Medicine**
*www.acsm.org*
P.O. Box 1440
Indianapolis, IN 46206
317–637–9200
317–634–7817 (fax)

For information about health and fitness.

**Diabetes Exercise & Sports Association (DESA)**
*www.diabetes-exercise.org*
8001 Montcastle Dr.
Nashville, TN 37221
800–898–4322
615–673–2077 (fax)
E-mail: desa@diabetes-exercise.org

For information and support for athletes and active people with diabetes.

**President's Council on Physical Fitness and Sports**
*www.fitness.gov*
Department W
200 Independence Ave., SW, Room 738-H
Washington, D.C. 20201
202–690–9000
202–690–5211 (fax)

For information about physical activity, exercise, and fitness.

# FOR PEOPLE OVER 50

**AARP Pharmacy Services**
*www.aarppharmacy.com*

Over-the-counter and prescription drugs delivered to your door in seven to 10 days. Competitive prices that are the same for members and nonmembers. May pay by credit card or be billed.

Mailing addresses and phone numbers vary based on plan selected. For more information, visit the website or contact AARP's main office.

601 E Street NW
Washington, D.C. 20049
1–888–OUR–AARP (1–888–687–2277)

**National Council on the Aging**
*www.ncoa.org*
1901 L Street, N.W.
4th floor
Washington, D.C. 20036
202–479–1200
202–479–0735 (fax)
E-mail: info@ncoa.org

Advocacy group concerned with developing and implementing high standards of care for the elderly. Referrals to local agencies concerned with the elderly.

# FOR EQUAL EMPLOYMENT INFORMATION

**American Bar Association—**
**Commission on Mental and Physical Disability Law**
*www.abanet.org/disability*
740 15th Street NW
Washington, D.C. 20005–1019
202–662–1000
202–662–1032 (fax)
E-mail: cmpdl@abanet.org

Provides information and technical assistance on all aspects of disability law.

**Disability Rights Education and Defense Fund, Inc. (DREDF)**
*www.dredf.org*
2212 6th Street
Berkeley, CA 94710
800–348–4232 (voice/TTY)
510–644–2555 (voice/TTY)
510–841–8645 (fax)
E-mail: info@dredf.org

Provides technical assistance and information to employers and individuals with disabilities on disability rights legislation and policies. Assists with legal representation.

**Equal Employment Opportunity Commission**
*www.eeoc.gov*
1801 L Street NW
Washington, D.C. 20507
202–663–4900
800–669–4000
202–663–4494 (TTY)
800–669–6820 (TTY)

National Dissemination Center for Children with Disabilities
*www.nichcy.org*
P.O. Box 1492
Washington, D.C. 20013
800–695–0285 (voice and TTY)
202–884–8441 (fax)
E-mail: nichcy@aed.org

Provides technical assistance and information on disabilities and disability-related issues.

# FOR HEALTH INSURANCE INFORMATION

### AARP Health Care Options
*www.aarphealth care.com*
800–317–8628 x712
800–232–7773 (TTY)

AARP administers a variety of health insurance plans, including personal health insurance plans, hospital plans, long-term care plans, Medicare Advantage plans, and supplemental plans. Plans are available to people 50 and over. Not all plans are available in all areas.

### Medicare Hot Line
*www.medicare.gov*
800–MEDICARE (800–633–4227)
877–486–2048 (TTY/TDD)
Centers for Medicare & Medicaid Services
7500 Security Boulevard
Baltimore MD 21244–1850

For information and various publications about Medicare.

**Social Security Administration**
*www.ssa.gov*
800–772–1213
800–325–0778 (TTY)
Social Security Administration
Office of Public Inquiries
Windsor Park Building
6401 Security Blvd.
Baltimore, MD 21235

For information and various publications about Medicare.

# AMERICAN DIABETES ASSOCIATION

**Community Offices**

**ALABAMA**
Birmingham 205–870–5172
Huntsville 256–539–4404

**ALASKA**
Anchorage 907–272–1424
Fairbanks 907–457–1557

**ARIZONA**
Phoenix 602–861–4731
Tucson 520–795–3711

**ARKANSAS**
Little Rock 501–221–7444

**CALIFORNIA**
Los Angeles 323–966–2890
Oceanside 619–754–9601
Sacramento 916–924–3232
San Diego 619–234–9897
San Francisco 510–654–4499
San Jose 408–241–1922
Santa Ana 714–662–7940

## COLORADO
Denver 720–855–1102

## CONNECTICUT
Middletown 203–639–0385

## DISTRICT OF COLUMBIA
Washington Metro 202–331–8303

## DELAWARE
Wilmington 302–656–0030

## FLORIDA
Fort Lauderdale 954–772–8040
Jacksonville 904–730–7200
Miami 305–477–8999
Orlando 407–660–1926
Pensacola 850–478–5957
Tampa 813–885–5007
West Palm Beach 561–689–2746

## GEORGIA
Atlanta 404–320–7100
Savannah 912–353–8110

## HAWAII
Honolulu 808–947–5979

## IDAHO
Boise 208–342–2774

## ILLINOIS
Bloomington 309–662–5955
Chicago 312–346–1805
Decatur 217–875–9011

## INDIANA
Evansville 812–476–6949
Indianapolis 317–352–9226

## IOWA
Cedar Rapids 319–247–5124

Davenport 515–276–2237
Des Moines 515–276–2237

**KANSAS**
Overland Park 913–383–8210
Wichita 316–684–6091

**KENTUCKY**
Lexington 859–268–9129
Louisville 502–452–6072

**LOUISIANA**
Baton Rouge 225–216–3980
Shreveport 318–425–2878

**MAINE**
Portland 207–774–7717

**MARYLAND**
Baltimore 410–265–0075
Salisbury 410–543–4530
Washington Metro 202–331–8303

**MASSACHUSETTS**
Boston 617–482–4580
Cape Cod 508–394–8818

**MICHIGAN**
Detroit 248–433–3830
Grand Rapids 616–458–9341

**MINNESOTA**
Bloomington 612–948–0236
Minneapolis 763–593–5333

**MISSOURI**
Kansas City 913–383–8210
Springfield 417–890–8400
St. Louis 314–822–5490

## MONTANA
Billings 406–256–0616

## NEBRASKA/SOUTH DAKOTA
Omaha 402–571–1101

## NEVADA
Las Vegas 702–369–9995

## NEW HAMPSHIRE
Manchester 603–627–9579

## NEW JERSEY
Cherry Hill 856–482–9047
Somerset 732–469–7979

## NEW MEXICO
Albuquerque 505–266–5716

## NEW YORK
Albany 518–218–1755
Amherst 716–835–0274
Hauppauge 631–348–0422
New York City 212–725–4925
Rochester 585–458–3040
Syracuse 315–438–8687
Utica 315–735–6434
White Plains 914–697–4987

## NORTH CAROLINA
Charlotte 704–373–9111
Raleigh 919–743–5400
Winston-Salem 336–472–9208

## NORTH DAKOTA
Fargo 701–234–0123

## OHIO
Akron 330–835–3149
Cincinnati 513–759–9330
Cleveland 216–328–9989
Columbus 614–436–1917
Toledo 419–841–5992

## OKLAHOMA
Oklahoma City 405–840–3881
Tulsa 918–492–3839

## OREGON
Eugene 541–343–0735
Portland 503–736–2770

## PENNSYLVANIA
Allentown 610–435–6700
Harrisburg 717–657–4310
Philadelphia 610–828–5003
Pittsburgh 412–824–1181

## RHODE ISLAND
Providence 401–351–0498

## SOUTH CAROLINA
Columbia 803–799–4246
Greenville 864–609–5054

## TENNESSEE
Knoxville 865–524–7868
Memphis 901–682–8232
Nashville 615–298–3066

## TEXAS
Amarillo 806–353–9219
Austin 512–472–9838
Corpus Christi 361–850–8778
Dallas 972–255–6900

Fort Worth 817–332–7110
Houston 713–977–7706
Lubbock 806–794–0691
McAllen 956–631–1118
Midland 432–570–1232
San Antonio 210–829–1765

**UTAH**
Salt Lake City 801–363–3024

**VERMONT**
Colchester 802–654–7716

**VIRGINIA**
Norfolk 757–424–6662
Richmond 804–225–8038
Washington Metro 202–331–8303

**WASHINGTON**
Everett 425–258–8116
Seattle 206–282–4616
Spokane 509–624–7478

**WEST VIRGINIA**
Charleston 304–768–2596

**WISCONSIN**
Madison 608–833–1060
Milwaukee 414–778–5500

# Index

# Other Titles from the American Diabetes Association

### Real-Life Guide to Diabetes
*by Hope S. Warshaw, MMSc, RD, CDE, BC-ADM,*
*and Joy Pape, RN, BSC, CDE, WOCN, CFCN*
*Real-Life Guide* puts everything you need to know
about diabetes into a one-of-a-kind book packed
with the information you won't find anywhere else.
Learn to prevent long-term complications, understand the ins and outs of health insurance, work
physical activity into your daily life, and control your
blood glucose, cholesterol, and blood pressure. Bring
a realistic approach to your diabetes care plan.
**Order no. 4893-01; Price $19.95**

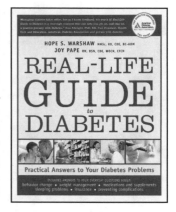

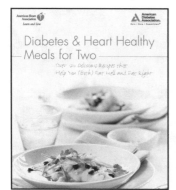

### Diabetes & Heart Healthy Meals for Two
*by the American Diabetes Association*
*and the American Heart Association*
If you or a loved one has diabetes, you need to
eat heart-healthy meals. The simple, flavorful recipes were designed for those looking to improve
or maintain their cardiovascular health. Each
recipe is for two people, making this book perfect for adults without children in the house or
for those who want to keep leftovers to a minimum. With over 170 recipes, there are countless
options to keep you heart at its healthiest and
your blood glucose under control.
**Order no. 4673-01; Price $18.95**

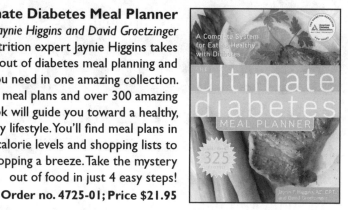
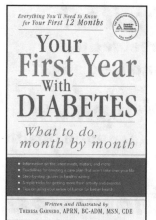

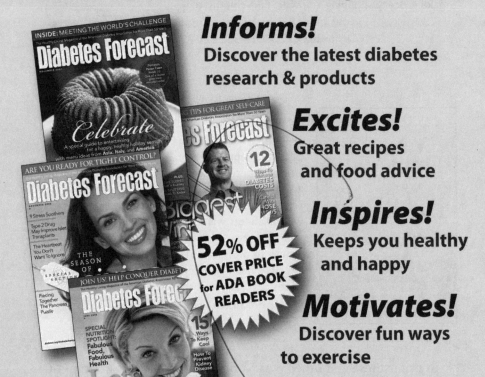